Soft Tissue Release

Hands-On Guides for Therapists

Jane Johnson, MCSP, MSc
The London Massage Company

Human Kinetics

Johnson, Jane, 1965-
   Soft tissue release / Jane Johnson.
      p. ; cm. -- (Hands-on guides for therapists)
   ISBN-13: 978-0-7360-7712-5 (soft cover : alk. paper)
   ISBN-10: 0-7360-7712-X (soft cover : alk. paper) 1. Massage
therapy. I. Title. II. Series: Hands-on guides for therapists.
   [DNLM: 1. Massage--methods. WB 537 J67s 2009]
   RM721.J645 2009
   615.8'22--dc22

                                                2008053144

ISBN-10: 0-7360-7712-X (print)   ISBN-10: 0-7360-8543-2 (Adobe PDF)
ISBN-13: 978-0-7360-7712-5 (print)   ISBN-13: 978-0-7360-8543-4 (Adobe PDF)

Copyright © 2009 by Jane Johnson

Acquisitions Editor: John Dickinson, PhD; **Developmental Editor:** Christine M. Drews; **Assistant Editor:** Katherine Maurer; **Copyeditor:** Ann Prisland; **Proofreader:** Darlene Rake; **Permission Manager:** Dalene Reeder; **Graphic Designer:** Nancy Rasmus; **Graphic Artist:** Dawn Sills; **Cover Designer:** Keith Blomberg ; **Photographer (cover and interior):** Neil Bernstein; **Photo Asset Manager:** Laura Fitch; **Visual Production Assistant:** Joyce Brumfield; **Photo Production Manager:** Jason Allen; **Art Manager:** Kelly Hendren; **Associate Art Manager:** Alan L. Wilborn; **Illustrators:** Jason M. McAlexander, MFA, and Tim Brummett; **Printer:** United Graphics

Special thanks to Douglas Nelson, LMT, for his expertise as the massage therapist in the photographs.

Printed in the United States of America   10 9 8 7 6 5 4 3 2 1

The paper in this book is certified under a sustainable forestry program.

Human Kinetics
Web site: www.HumanKinetics.com

United States: Human Kinetics
P.O. Box 5076
Champaign, IL 61825-5076
800-747-4457
e-mail: humank@hkusa.com

Canada: Human Kinetics
475 Devonshire Road Unit 100
Windsor, ON N8Y 2L5
800-465-7301 (in Canada only)
e-mail: info@hkcanada.com

Europe: Human Kinetics
107 Bradford Road
Stanningley
Leeds LS28 6AT, United Kingdom
+44 (0) 113 255 5665
e-mail: hk@hkeurope.com

Australia: Human Kinetics
57A Price Avenue
Lower Mitcham, South Australia 5062
08 8372 0999
e-mail: info@hkaustralia.com

New Zealand: Human Kinetics
Division of Sports Distributors NZ Ltd.
P.O. Box 300 226 Albany
North Shore City
Auckland
0064 9 448 1207
e-mail: info@humankinetics.co.nz

*To my son, Jake Johnson, whose inquiring mind is
a constant reminder of the need to ask questions
and the value of experimentation.*

Contents

PART III Applying Soft Tissue Release

PART IV Soft Tissue Release Programmes

Series Preface

Massage may be one of the oldest therapies still used today. At present more therapists than ever before are practicing an ever-expanding range of massage techniques. Many of these techniques are taught through massage schools and within degree courses. Our need now is to provide the best clinical and educational resources that will enable massage therapists to learn the required techniques for delivering massage therapy to clients. Human Kinetics has developed the Hands-On Guides for Therapists series with this in mind.

The Hands-On Guides for Therapists series provides specific tools of assessment and treatment that fall well within the realm of massage therapists but may also be useful for other bodyworkers, such as osteopaths and fitness instructors. Each book in the series is a step-by-step guide to delivering the techniques to clients. Each book features a full-colour interior packed with photos illustrating every technique. Tips provide handy advice to help you adjust your technique, and the Client Talk boxes contain examples of how the techniques can be used with clients who have particular problems. Throughout each book are questions that enable you to test your knowledge and skill, which will be particularly helpful if you are attempting to pass a qualification exam. We've even provided the answers too!

You might be using a book from the Hands-On Guides for Therapists series to obtain the required skills to help you pass a course or to brush up on skills you learned in the past. You might be a course tutor looking for ways to make massage therapy come alive with your students. This series provides easy-to-follow steps that will make the transition from theory to practice seem effortless. The Hands-On Guides for Therapists series is an essential resource for all those who are serious about massage therapy.

Preface

This book has been written for all therapists wishing to add to their existing soft tissue skills. It has been designed so that it may be used as a stand-alone text, the photographs helping to support the step-by-step explanations, but it may be equally valuable when used as a support text for those taking workshops in soft tissue release (STR) or studying on longer courses where STR forms one of the modules. Many therapists already trained in the use of STR may find it a helpful reference. As this form of stretching may also be performed through clothing, fitness instructors, sport coaches, sport therapists, physiotherapists, osteopaths, chiropractors and other bodyworkers may also find this book beneficial.

Part I introduces the basics of soft tissue release, including how the technique works, who it may benefit, safety considerations and a brief description of the three methods of applying STR. Part II then provides instructions for applying the three methods—passive (chapter 3), active-assisted (chapter 4) and active (chapter 5). It includes condensed instructions and one representative photo for each stretch. In part III, each stretch is explained and illustrated in full and the chapters are organized by body part: chapter 6 contains stretches for the muscles of the trunk, chapter 7 the lower limbs and chapter 8 the upper limbs. Finally, part IV includes a comprehensive chapter on client consultation and designing individualised STR programmes.

There are three ways you could use this book. First, you could concentrate on learning the three different forms of STR, passive, active-assisted and active, described in chapters 3, 4 and 5. Second, you could practice applying STR by body part, working through chapter 6 for the trunk, chapter 7 for the lower limbs and chapter 8 for the upper limbs. Alternatively, you could look through the photo index at the end of the book. Here you will find thumbnail images grouping STR according to the position of the client—prone, supine, side lying and sitting.

Available as an E-BOOK at www.HumanKinetics.com

As you will discover, there are many different ways to apply STR. I hope that you will experiment with them all in order to find the ones that work best for you. Massage therapy is a vibrant, dynamic profession that gains from collaboration and discussion. Please feel free to send comments, enquiries and suggestions to me.

Acknowledgements

I am indebted to the many people who helped with the completion of this book. Thank you to John Dickinson, acquisitions editor at Human Kinetics, for accepting my original proposal and helping to formulate the final structure of the book; to Christine Drews, instrumental in shaping and finalizing the text; to Kate Maurer for her vigilant checking of both text and photographs; and to Nancy Rasmus for her wonderfully clear graphic design.

I would also like to thank the photographer, Neil Bernstein, and massage therapist, Douglas Nelson, LMT, who together have captured the essence of soft tissue release with its many different forms. This would not have been possible if it were not also for our models, Laura Czys, Gregg Henness, Melinda Lin-Roberts and Patrick Mustain, on whom the techniques are demonstrated.

Finally, I would like to thank the many students and workshop attendees I have met and continue to meet, who over the years have helped inform my practice with their enthusiasm for soft tissue techniques.

PART I

Getting Started With Soft Tissue Release

Welcome to *Soft Tissue Release*. In this first part of the book you will find everything necessary to help you get started with this great technique. In chapter 1 you will learn about the kinds of clients for whom STR is appropriate, how the technique works, the kinds of settings in which it can be performed, its benefits and the kinds of conditions for which it is helpful. Chapter 2 provides information about useful equipment, the importance of the client consultation, simple safety points and a brief description of the three methods of applying STR. Also covered in this chapter are ideas for measuring the effectiveness of STR as well as answers to frequently asked questions and lots of troubleshooting tips, useful to refer back to as you work through the book. At the end of these and each subsequent chapter you will discover some quick questions, which you may wish to answer to determine your level of understanding.

Introduction to Soft Tissue Release

Popularly known as STR, soft tissue release is an advanced massage technique widely used in assessing and stretching soft tissues. Soft tissues include muscle fibres, their tendons and the deep and superficial fascia surrounding and invaginating these tissues. Stretching is often used for easing the pain of muscle tension and realigning the body so that it functions in a more optimal way. However, unlike generalized stretching, soft tissue release targets specific areas of tension within a muscle. It is also useful for targeting muscles that are difficult to stretch actively (the fibularis muscle group, or peroneals, for example) and for isolating a muscle within a group of muscles that would normally stretch together (the vastus lateralis from the quadriceps, for example). It has proven useful in the treatment of certain conditions such as medial and lateral epicondylitis and plantar fasciitis, perhaps because it stimulates tissue repair in these conditions.

Who Should Have Soft Tissue Release?

Almost anyone will benefit from soft tissue release. It is particularly useful for the following people:

- Anyone who takes part in sports or exercise. Those taking part in a regular stretching programme will benefit from STR. It is useful before an event when time is limited and the athlete wants to target specific areas of tension; in this case, STR may be applied in a light and brisk manner. Between events it is useful as an assessment tool for identifying tightness in tissues that may limit performance.

- Anyone recovering from a musculoskeletal injury. Soft tissues shorten, atrophy and weaken as a result of immobility. Used correctly, STR may help to lengthen and encourage pliability in tight tissues. In this way it helps a client regain range of motion in a joint. Active stretching is known to help with the orientation of collagen fibres during healing.

- Anyone who maintains a static posture for long periods. Office workers and drivers who remain seated for long periods often have neck and shoulder pain due to increased muscle tension. STR may be used for alleviating neck pain associated with static postures.

- Anyone seeking treatment for lateral epicondylitis, medial epicondylitis or plantar fasciitis. It is also used as an adjunct in the treatment of shin splints and tight hamstrings. Applying STR to the pectorals is helpful for overcoming kyphotic postures.

- Anyone needing treatment for increased muscle tension and for old scar tissue. Such areas are palpable, and STR provides the therapist with an additional massage tool to help stretch and realign areas of soft tissue popularly described as being congested.

- Anyone who needs treatment of trigger points (localized muscle fibres believed to be in an unhealthy state of contraction and tender to the touch).

How Does Soft Tissue Release Work?

Take a look at the pictures shown here. They represent what happens when a gross stretch is applied to a muscle. The therapist is holding two resistance bands tied together, one red, the other black. The red resistance band is extremely stretchy; the black is tough and less stretchy. The red resistance band represents normal, healthy muscle tissue. The black resistance band represents an area of tight muscle tissue. Together these represent one whole muscle. Look at what happens in figure 1.1 when the therapist moves his right hand. Which part of the muscle does the stretching: the pliable (red) part or the tough (black) part? Clearly, the pliable band is doing the most stretching.

Now look at figure 1.2. What happens when the therapist moves his left hand? Which part of the muscle stretches the most: the pliable (red) part or the tough (black) part? Again, the pliable band is doing most of the stretching.

And finally, notice what happens when the therapist moves both his right and left hands apart so they are equidistant (figure 1.3).

You can see from these illustrations that it is the pliable part of the muscle (the red band in these illustrations) that does most of the stretching, irrespective of which end of the muscle is moved. To target the less pliable part of the muscle—the area of palpable tightness—you need to localize the stretch. This is exactly what STR does.

To localize the stretch, you need to 'fix' part of the muscle against underlying structures to create a false insertion point. The fixing—described throughout this book as a *lock*—prevents some parts of the muscle from moving and is achieved when a therapist uses his or her own upper body or a massage tool. When a muscle is stretched, its insertion points are moved apart from one another—that is, the area of tissue between the insertion points stretches. Creating false insertion points results in a more intense stretch in some parts of the muscle.

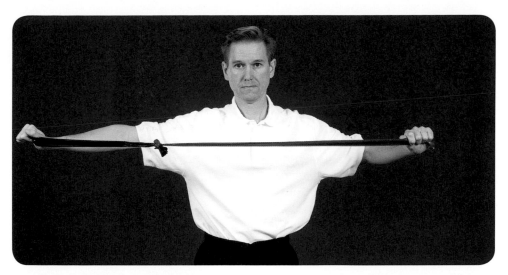

Figure 1.1 Notice which band is doing the stretching.

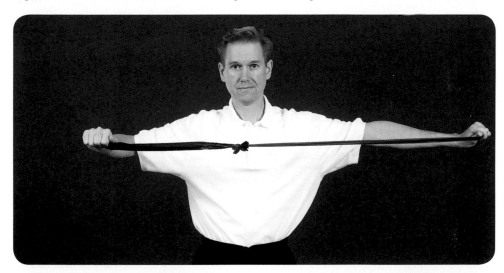

Figure 1.2 Which band is doing the stretching now?

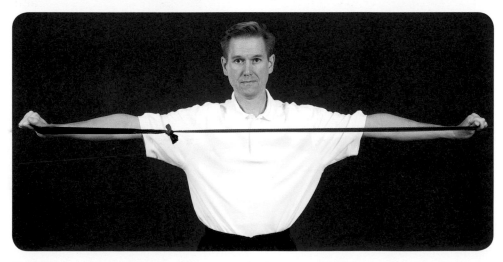

Figure 1.3 Even with an equidistant stretch, the more pliable band does the most stretching.

Look at figure 1.4, which is an illustration of the soleus. You probably already know that the soleus originates from the posterior shaft of the tibia and inserts into the calcaneus. If you pull up your toes (dorsiflexing your foot and ankle), this stretches the muscles of the calf (which are the plantar flexors). Dorsiflexion is therefore a way of applying a gross stretch to the soleus.

Now look at figure 1.5. Imagine locking the muscle to the tibia slightly distal (Lock A) to its actual origin. Can you see that if you were to stretch the muscle now, only those fibres running from the new origin (A) to the calcaneus would be able to stretch? Would you agree that, providing you are able to dorsiflex through the *same* range of motion as in the first stretch, greater force has been placed on those fibres being stretched? This occurs because the small amount of muscle tissue superior to lock A is no longer being stretched.

Now look at figure 1.6. A second imaginary origin (Lock B) for the soleus is even more distal on the tibia, broadly locking it to the underlying structures. Performing a stretch now will place even greater tension on the stretching fibres than if the lock had remained at (A).

Finally, you could create a third false origin (Lock C) yet more distal to the actual origin (see figure 1.7). In this example only the most distal portion of the soleus stretches when the foot and ankle are dorsiflexed.

In reality it is not possible—or advisable—to lock the entire breadth of the muscle, but this is the principle behind how STR works.

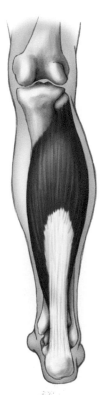

Figure 1.4 The soleus.

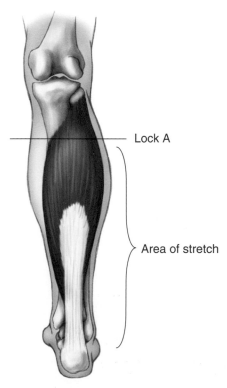

Figure 1.5 Locking the soleus muscle slightly distal to its actual origin (Lock A).

An alternative is to apply a specific rather than a broad lock, for example on the biceps brachii, as illustrated in figure 1.8. The areas of muscle fibre distal to each of the locks are put under greater stretch each time the elbow is extended. To understand this concept of a specific stretch, think of muscle fibres as the strings

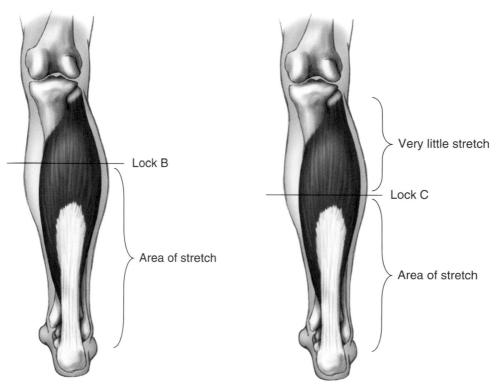

Lock B

Area of stretch

Very little stretch

Lock C

Area of stretch

Figure 1.6 Locking the soleus more distal on the tibia (Lock B).

Figure 1.7 Locking the soleus even more distal on the tibia (Lock C).

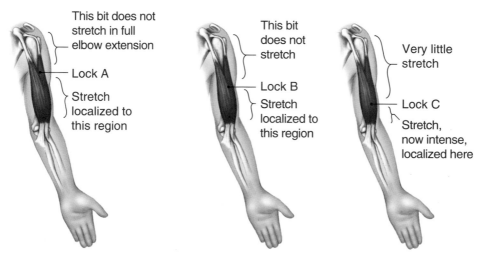

This bit does not stretch in full elbow extension

Lock A

Stretch localized to this region

This bit does not stretch

Lock B

Stretch localized to this region

Very little stretch

Lock C

Stretch, now intense, localized here

Figure 1.8 In applying specific locks, the areas of muscle fibre distal to each of the locks are put under greater stretch each time the elbow is extended.

of a guitar: Placing your finger across all of the strings, as in the previous example of the soleus, is quite different from placing your finger across one string, as in the case of using your elbow to apply a lock to the biceps. For a start, it is quite difficult to exert the same pressure across all strings that you would use to fix just one string. When playing the guitar, if you use the tip and pad of your finger to fix just one string, with one specific lock, only that string is affected, yet it is affected intensely. However, if you use more of your finger in an attempt to make a lock across all of the strings, you affect all of the strings when you play, though perhaps not as intensely.

Where Can Soft Tissue Release Take Place?

Soft tissue release can be used anywhere because it may be performed through clothing or a towel and in prone, supine or seated positions.

■   *In the office.* When working at a computer or with other office equipment, office workers may find it useful to apply active STR to their wrist and finger flexors and extensors.

■   *Whilst seated.* STR can be applied actively to the soles of the feet using a spiky ball or foot roller. STR may also be applied actively to the quadriceps when sitting. Therapists who provide seated, on-site massage may benefit from incorporating STR to the levator scapulae and the upper trapezius.

■   *In the park.* STR to the hamstrings and tibialis anterior can be performed in the park or by the side of a running track.

■   *On the tennis court.* After a match, STR to wrist and finger extensors can provide temporary relief from the discomfort of lateral epicondylitis (tennis elbow).

■   *On the golf course.* STR may provide temporary relief from medial epicondylitis (golfer's elbow).

■   *By the pool.* By working through a towel and taking care to keep the client warm, a therapist may apply STR to all major muscle groups.

■   *In the clinic.* STR can be performed as part of a holistic massage treatment, or it could form an entire treatment session in itself. Clinic sessions are useful when working with sensitive areas such as the iliacus because the client needs to be comfortable and relaxed.

■   *At home.* Almost anyone can follow a home stretching programme using simple tools to apply a gentle lock into soft tissues.

When Should Soft Tissue Release Be Done?

When performed slowly and conscientiously, soft tissue release may be used before, during or after a massage treatment or as a treatment in itself. Soft tissue becomes more pliable when warm, and most forms of stretching may be more effective when applied to warm tissues. However, increases in joint range are also attainable when STR is applied to tissues that have not been warmed. It is a perfectly safe form of stretching, providing movements are slow and controlled.

Stretching decreases muscle force and should therefore be used with caution in a pre-event setting. In this case it could help increase range of motion in joints, as long as care is taken not to overstretch the associated muscles. It may be valuable in helping to overcome excessive tightness or spasming in localized areas of tissue that need immediate attention before a sporting event.

When using STR in a post-event setting, take care not to work too deeply. There may be microtrauma to tissues, so it is best to use STR conservatively as an assessment tool and save deeper work for part of a maintenance massage. Also, after excessive exercise or training, increased levels of pain-relieving hormones may decrease a client's perception of pain, and as a result, a client may be less able to give accurate feedback relating to the degree of pressure he or she is sensing. In both pre- and post-event work, STR tends to be used as an adjunct to other forms of treatment for overcoming cramping and for maintaining muscle length. Between training sessions and as part of some forms of rehabilitation, it may be used as a form of deep, intense stretching.

Overall, STR should be used when there is a reason to use it! This reason could be simply because the client likes the sensation of STR or because as a therapist you have identified areas of tension that need to be addressed. It is unlikely that you will be working with the same client on a daily basis unless the client is preparing for or involved in an ongoing sporting event. STR can certainly be used weekly, and perhaps two or three times a week, on the same muscle. Use your own judgement to ensure you do not overwork an area. Once STR has been applied two or three times to a muscle within a treatment session, the muscle will be noticeably more pliable.

Benefits of Soft Tissue Release

Soft tissue release is used for a variety of reasons, perhaps most commonly because it stretches soft tissues. It is therefore beneficial because it improves flexibility and posture, alleviates the pain of muscle tension and takes pressure off associated joint structures. It helps maintain or increase range of motion within a joint and, combined with excellent palpation skills, helps therapists assess the degree of tension within and between soft tissues. Many clients also enjoy the sensation of STR and are happy to have it incorporated into their massage routines. It provides therapists with another tool they can employ and may thus help keep massage routines varied. STR is especially useful in clinical settings where clients need to stretch muscles but cannot take joints through a full range of motion. For example, after many forms of knee surgery, patients are encouraged to flex and extend their knees to maintain joint integrity and pliability of surrounding tissue. Movement is believed to facilitate the healing process but is often limited due to pain and swelling. Used at the right juncture in treatment, STR can help in stretching the tissues without causing the joint to move through its full range; for example, STR can be applied to the quadriceps with the client flexing the knee to only 90 degrees. STR is particularly useful as part of the rehabilitation process when used for achieving small increases in range that might not otherwise be possible.

CLIENT TALK

I used STR to the quadriceps of a client who had been in a full-length leg cast and, because of tightening of the knee joint capsule, was initially unable to gain full knee flexion. We started cautiously, gaining very small increases in joint range initially, combining STR with massage in an attempt to stimulate the quadriceps. I had to hold the client's leg in extension and lower it passively because he did not have strength in his quadriceps to do this. I learned that passive STR to the quadriceps is actually quite strenuous for the therapist, and I had to take great care not to strain my back whilst performing it.

Closing Remarks

You have learned that soft tissue release targets specific areas of tension in a muscle. It especially stretches soft tissues: muscle fibres, their tendons and the fascia. It is safe and effective for most people.

Now that you have an idea of what STR is, how it works, who could receive it and when and where it can be used, you are ready to discover more about the various ways of locking muscles and using massage tools. Plus you are ready to learn lots of tips and tricks to get started on the right track in using this technique as well as ideas for measuring your effectiveness.

Quick Questions

1. How does STR differ from generalized stretching?
2. Give three examples of how a muscle might be locked.
3. When applying a lock, do you start at the proximal or distal end of the muscle?
4. Why should STR be used cautiously in a pre-event setting?
5. Why should deep STR be avoided in a post-event setting?

Preparing for Soft Tissue Release

In this chapter, you'll learn the basics of STR: various methods of locking tissues, including their advantages and disadvantages; types of massage tools; potential safety issues; and an overview of the three types of STR: passive, active-assisted and active. At the end of the chapter, you'll find frequently asked questions and troubleshooting tips, as well as a section on measuring the effectiveness of your treatments. You'll have everything you need to get started with this versatile stretching technique.

Equipment Required

Soft tissue release may be applied without any equipment at all. The therapist locks the client's muscles using his or her own upper limb. However, in some cases, using tools to help lock and stretch the muscles may be desirable.

Using Your Body to Apply STR

Your upper body provides a surprising array of options for applying STR. Forearms can provide broad locks, and elbows can provide localized locks; similarly, each part of the upper limb can be used for unique purposes. Massage therapists are notorious for sustaining upper limb injuries due to overuse. These can easily be avoided by using your forearms, fists and elbows using the suggestions provided here.

FOREARM   Forearms are used on large, bulky muscles, such as the quadriceps, calf muscles and gluteals. Your forearm provides a strong, broad lock, good for providing overall stretch and for use with clients who cannot tolerate a more specific lock. These locks are easy to apply, and the amount of contact with the client's muscles can be varied—a forearm lock to the quadriceps is broad, whereas a lock to the calf is a

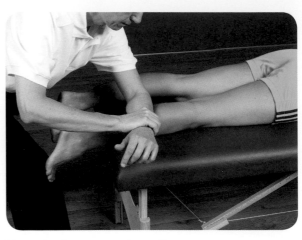

Using the forearm on the calf.

little more specific. Even though forearm locks create more leverage and are safer for the therapist's own joints, some therapists avoid these locks, claiming they find it difficult to assess tissues without using their hands. It is worth practicing STR using your forearms in order to avoid potential overuse injuries. The disadvantage of using your forearms is that they provide a less specific stretch than your elbow does, and forearms are difficult to use on small muscle groups.

ELBOW   Elbows are used in applying firm, deep pressure, which locks tissues in such a way as to direct the stretch to the tight parts of the muscle. Elbows are good for working large, bulky muscles, especially when a client wants to stretch a muscle actively or where there is palpable tightness, perhaps resulting from scar tissue. Elbows are also useful for targeting strap-like muscles, such as the levator scapulae, or on muscles that would not be properly locked with the use of forearms due to their location, such as tibialis anterior and fibularis (peroneal) muscles. Using an elbow to lock tissues does not necessitate the application of force. With practice, elbows may be used sensitively on levator scapulae and around the upper fibres of the trapezius in order to provide a localized lock.

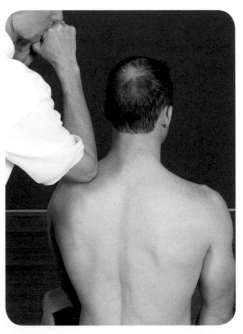

Using the elbow on the levator scapula.

SOFT FISTS Sometimes it is necessary to provide a broad lock, but there is not enough room for your forearm or hands. Using cupped fingers and applying a soft fist works well on pectorals. You can use the pads of your fingers, but the fingers might press into the ribs, which would be uncomfortable for the client because the pectorals are strong and need a fairly firm lock.

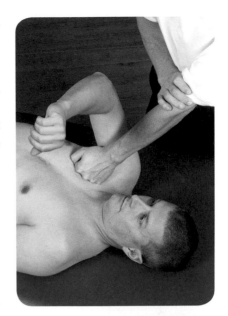

Using soft fists on the pectorals.

SINGLE FIST To work an area more specifically than with a forearm, but less specifically than with an elbow, you could use a single fist. This technique works well on the small area of the rhomboids and when working the hamstrings of a client for the first time to gauge resistance in the tissues.

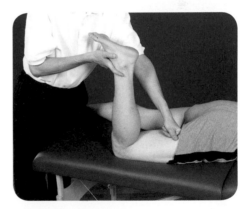

Using a single fist on the hamstrings.

PALM Palms provide a flat surface for a lock but place some stress on the therapist's wrist joint, so they should be used with care. Because palm pressure is not deep, it is good for providing a gentle lock, which is useful for the application of mild STR before or after sporting events.

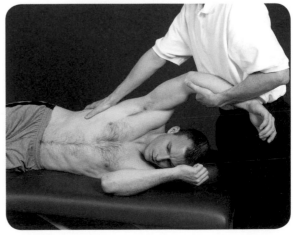

Using palms on the latissimus dorsi.

GRIP   Sometimes simply gripping the muscle can be a way of providing a lock. Gripping works best on small biceps and triceps that do not require a great degree of stretch. To avoid pinching the muscle, simply apply some oil and grip through a facecloth or small towel.

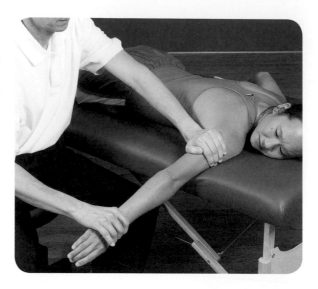

Gripping the triceps.

REINFORCED THUMBS   These are used in locking specific areas of muscle, generally smaller muscles that do not require much force for a lock. Reinforced thumbs work well on the common flexor and extensor origins of the wrist. If you discover that you need to apply a lot of pressure through your thumbs, then change the form of lock you are using. Practice applying gentle pressure through your forearms or elbow rather than risk damaging your thumb joints. This may necessitate positioning the client in a seated position to receive STR.

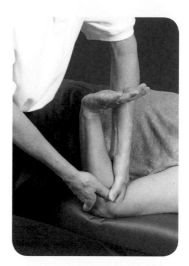

Using reinforced thumbs on the wrist extensors.

SINGLE THUMB   Thumbs must be used with caution and only to lock tissues when gentle pressure is required. Overuse of thumbs during treatment is a common cause of injury for massage therapists. Wherever possible, use an alternative method of locking.

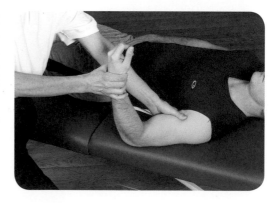

Using a single thumb on the biceps.

FINGERS   It is useful to use fingers to lock sensitive tissues, such as the scalene muscles, that require very little pressure. Fingers may also be useful in applying STR to the iliacus, and they may be cupped for reinforcement.

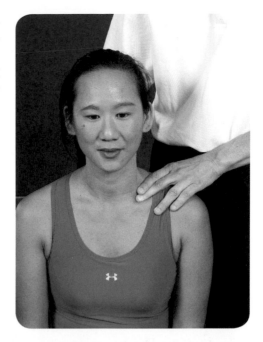

Using fingers on the scalenes.

KNUCKLES   Knuckles are useful for applying a lock to erector spinae muscles and are a good alternative to thumbs. As with the application of all forms of STR, it is important to keep your knuckle lock static. Avoid *worrying* the tissues, or rubbing them in a friction-like manner, because this simply grinds your knuckle joints.

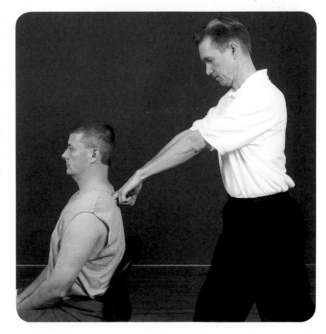

Using knuckles on the erector spinae.

Using Tools to Apply STR

As with the application of all forms of therapy, you need to protect your own body when working. Fortunately, STR may be applied safely and effectively if certain guidelines are followed, and a variety of tools provide additional support. Shown here is a selection of tools designed for use in bodywork as well as some objects that have been improvised for this purpose.

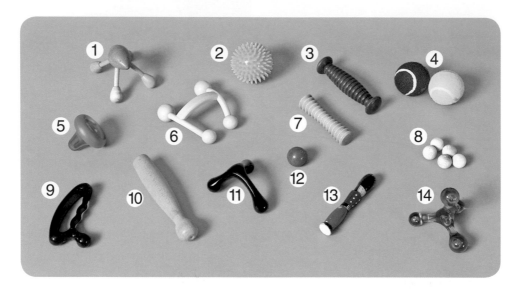

1 Wooden 'mouse'

2 Plastic therapy ball with spikes

3 Wooden foot roller (convex)

4 Tennis-type balls from a pet shop

5 The Knobble massage tool

6 Hard plastic Quad Nobber

7 Wooden foot roller (concave), also used on forearms

8 Wooden spheres from a hardware store

9 Index Knobber

10 Child's wooden skittle from a thrift shop

11 Hard plastic massage tool

12 Plastic high-bounce ball (soft) from a toy shop

13 Child's wooden toy soldier

14 Plastic Jacknobber

Shown here is an Index Knobber being used in treating the sole of the foot. It could work equally well on any area that required deep, localized pressure; it makes a good alternative to using your thumb.

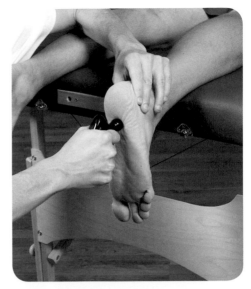

Index Knobber to sole of foot.

The spiky therapy balls are useful for applying active STR to the soles of the feet when sitting. Quad Nobbers can be used on the quadriceps and also work well on the erector spinae as an alternative to knuckles.

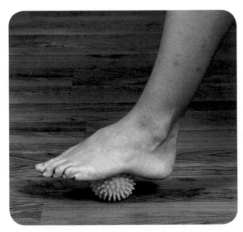

Spiky ball to sole of foot.

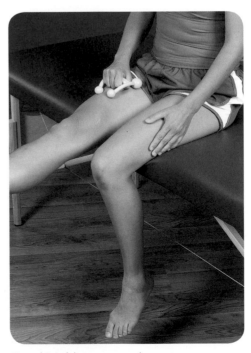

Quad Nobber on quads.

The tennis-type balls are actually for dogs and deform much less readily than regular tennis balls. They are useful for applying active STR to hamstrings or quadriceps as shown here.

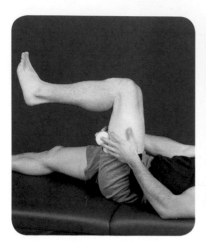
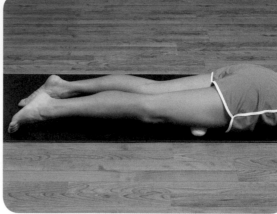

Tennis-type ball to hamstrings.   Tennis-type ball to quadriceps.

Other pieces of useful equipment include a facecloth or small towel and some massage oil. STR can be applied through clothing, but for a stronger lock, apply oil to the client's skin and work through a facecloth or small towel.

Consultation With the Client

As with all forms of therapy, when you meet a client for the first time, start with an initial client consultation in which you discover the nature of your client's problem and what he or she hopes to gain from your treatment. Take a detailed history, making note of any medication the client is taking, and identify whether there are any contraindications to your treatment plan. Then carry out a physical assessment, which will vary depending on what it is you will be treating. For example, in assessing someone who has come to you because he or she still has a stiff joint from an old ankle sprain, you will need to test the ankle's range of motion; if you are dealing with an office worker who has neck pain, you may want to do a seated postural assessment (and not touch the ankles at all). At the end of your consultation, you will likely set out the aims of your treatment (e.g., to alleviate pain, increase range of motion, reduce muscle stiffness from exercise training), if necessary describing these in lay terms to ensure your client is in agreement with what you aim to do and hope to achieve. Chapter 9 covers the topic of client consultation in detail, with suggested questions, possible physical assessments and methods of documentation.

Caution and Safety Issues

Soft tissue release is a form of assisted stretching that is safe and effective for the majority of clients. There is a simple rule when deciding whether or not a client may receive soft tissue release: If you would not normally treat the client with massage, bodywork or stretching, the client should not receive STR.

Because the technique involves gentle pressure into soft tissue, exercise caution when applying it to clients who bruise easily or who have thin skin. When treating clients who are hypermobile (increased range of motion in the joints, common amongst professional dancers, for example) consider whether stretching the tissues, and thus improving joint range, is actually desirable. Soft tissue release is not suitable for clients with hypermobility syndromes because there may be excessive stretch in the pliability of tissues.

When first receiving a lock, most clients feel no stretch at all. It is not until the lock nears the distal end of the muscle that the stretch intensifies. If you happen to lock a trigger spot, the client will report slight discomfort. This discomfort should be expressed in terms of being 'comfortably tolerable' or 'it hurts, but it feels good'. If you are a massage therapist, you are probably familiar with such statements. However, if the client reports that the sensation has become truly uncomfortable, you should not perform STR. It may be that there is some underlying inflammation not yet palpable. A simple rule is that the feeling of increased localized tension should dissipate within about a minute of applying a lock. If it does not, remove the lock. This feeling is quite unlike that of old scar tissue, which is palpably tight but causes no discomfort.

Although rare, clients sometimes report feeling sore after STR, as with some other forms of stretching. The feeling has been likened to delayed onset muscle soreness (DOMS). For this reason, you should avoid overworking any one particular area and aim to incorporate STR with oil massage if possible. Theoretically, massage between sessions of STR helps flush fresh blood into tissues and improve muscle health. Some therapists like to warn clients that in rare cases soreness may occur but will resolve itself within about 12 hours. However, others argue that this sets up a self-fulfilling prophecy and promotes the likelihood that the client will experience that exact soreness.

Pre- and post-event STR should not be applied too deeply. Before an event, it could decrease muscle power and may also be deeply relaxing. Pre-event STR should be used in an upbeat manner and with the aim of invigorating the client and maintaining joint range. Post-event STR may increase the likelihood of bruising after microtrauma to tissues. Post-event STR should be used generally and to help overcome cramping.

As a therapist, you should avoid overusing your upper limbs when applying any technique, including STR. Wherever possible, transfer your body weight through your forearms and elbows or use a massage tool as an alternative to using your thumbs. Save your thumbs and fingers for delicate work on smaller, more pliable tissues. To get even more leverage, try working with your treatment couch an inch or two lower than you have it at present. Practice leaning in to your client, transferring your weight to their tissues. Many therapists adopt the position of leaning in but actually use a lot of energy holding the leaning-in stance because they are fearful of hurting the client. Make it your intention to create locks by gently but firmly leaning in towards your client *before* beginning treatment. By working slowly and conscientiously, you will discover that with practice, STR is a powerful, safe and effective tool for stretching soft tissues.

Three Methods of STR

Soft tissue release may be performed in three ways: passive, active-assisted or active (see the examples on p. 21).

1. *Passive*. When STR is performed passively, the therapist applies a lock and moves the client's body part so as to facilitate a stretch.
2. *Active-assisted*. This form of STR requires the client and therapist to work together. Usually, the therapist applies a lock, and the client moves his or her body part to bring about the stretch.
3. *Active*. In active STR, the client applies a lock to himself or herself and also performs the stretch without assistance. Active STR can be performed by almost anyone and does not require a therapist be present.

Throughout this book we use common anatomical language. However, clients are unlikely to understand these terms unless they are therapists or health professionals themselves. It takes practice to explain to clients what they are required to do for active-assisted STR without using technical language. Many clients may not understand what you mean if you ask them to invert or evert a foot, for example, or to flex or extend a wrist. One tip is to demonstrate the action you require before making your lock. If you want to give the command of 'up' or 'down' when referring to a wrist movement, for example, then you need to demonstrate what you mean by those commands. Another tip is to avoid mixing different types of STR within the same treatment. If you start with active-assisted STR, a client may think he or she is required to assist throughout a treatment and may not relax when you want to perform passive STR. However, many clients soon become accustomed to STR and will demonstrate a preference for whether they want to take part (active-assisted) or whether they prefer to receive the treatment passively.

Measuring the Effectiveness of STR

It is useful to have a benchmark against which to measure whether a treatment has been effective. This is equally true of STR. Here are some ideas to help you measure the effectiveness of STR.

Using Wrist Flexors to Compare the Three Types of STR

PASSIVE STR   The therapist locks the common flexor origin with the client's wrist in flexion and then moves the wrist into extension.

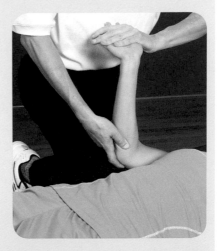

ACTIVE-ASSISTED STR   The therapist locks the client's common flexor origin, then asks the client to extend her wrist actively.

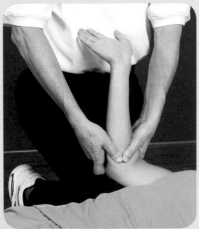

ACTIVE STR   The client locks her own common flexor origin and then extends her wrist.

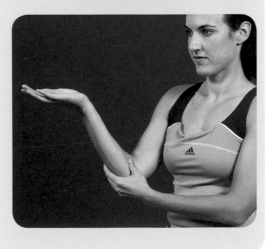

- *Pain*. If STR is being used to alleviate the discomfort of muscle tension, one of the easiest methods for measuring effectiveness is simply to use self-reporting measures. Not surprisingly, most clients feel better after massage and report feeling less discomfort, whether this was initially described as pain, pulling, cramping or aching. Most therapists are familiar with asking clients how they feel after treatment.

- *Visual analogue scale (VAS)*. This is simply a horizontal line onto which two extremes have been written. One extreme could be 'no discomfort' and the other extreme could be 'worst discomfort ever!' Before and after treatment, ask the client to mark the scale according to how he or she is feeling. (You can see examples of visual analogue scales in figures 9.4 and 9.8, pages 141 and 151.) A VAS is useful for measuring subjective descriptors such as pain or stiffness.

- *Movement tests*. If STR has been applied to help increase range of motion in a joint, you could do tests such as the straight leg raise (for hamstrings). Measure the straight leg raise before and after applying STR to the hamstrings and record whether there has been any increase in range at the hip joint as a result of your treatment. A simple test for quadriceps flexibility is the prone knee bend: ask the client to flex his or her knee while in a prone position; observe how close the client's foot comes to the buttock on that side. After treatment to lengthen the quadriceps, the client should be able to reach his or her foot closer to the buttock than before treatment (make sure the client avoids excessive lordosis in the lower back).

- *Sit-and-reach test*. A simple way to measure the effectiveness of active STR to the hamstrings is to ask your client to reach forward and try to touch his or her toes. Notice how far the client can reach and ask what sensations are felt in the hamstring muscles. Spend five to seven minutes applying STR to the hamstrings, then retest the client. Was the client able to touch his or her toes more easily? Did the client have less tightness in the hamstring muscles? (This test also tests flexibility in the muscles of the back and should not be performed by clients who have recently suffered trauma to the lumbar spine.)

Frequently Asked Questions and Troubleshooting Tips

How long should I hold my lock at the end of the stretch?

Once the tissues are stretched, remove the lock.

How much pressure should I apply when locking in?

Enough to lock the tissues. If this causes discomfort to the client or to you, read the troubleshooting tips on the next page.

Should I encourage the client to tolerate pain?

Never. STR should be comfortable. Clients should feel a mild stretch, but this may vary depending on which part of the muscle you are working.

How many times should I perform STR to one muscle?

You may find that for large muscles, such as hamstrings, you need to work all over them in lines, from proximal to distal, to cover the tissues adequately. Once you have done each line three times, both you and the client should sense the tissues have stretched. Overall, you need to avoid overworking one muscle group. Sometimes it is a good idea to apply STR two or three times, move to a different part of the body, then return to the original STR site and check to see whether both you and the client perceive the tissue to have stretched.

If after working through this book you are still having difficulty applying STR, here are some things you can try:

- If you can't seem to get a grip on the soft tissue, practice changing your lock. Have you tried using the flat of your palm or a soft fist, forearm, elbow or knuckles? An alternative is to apply a small amount of oil onto the skin, then work through a towel. The towel will grip the oil and provide a stronger lock.

- If the lock is uncomfortable for the client, try using less pressure. Try working through clothing or a small towel to dissipate your lock. Alternatively, make sure you are not on bone. This is a common mistake people make when first learning to apply STR to the rhomboids: avoid pressing into the medial border of the scapulae. When working the pectorals, avoid pressing perpendicularly into the ribs. Check that you are not pressing into a nerve plexus, which can cause a tingling sensation for the client. Check that you are not pulling on the skin too hard.

- If your client does not seem to feel the stretch, try adding more pressure. To increase pressure, use your elbows or forearms and lean into the lock. Alternatively, make sure you take up the slack in the soft tissues before performing the stretch. Check that you are directing your pressure towards the proximal end of the limb. Many clients do not experience much of a stretch with passive STR. If this is the case, try using active STR and see what happens.

- If it is uncomfortable for you to apply the lock with your fingers, hands or thumbs, try using a massage tool. Always aim to protect your own joints. If you still can't apply the lock comfortably, don't do it at all.

- If you can't seem to get comfortable yourself, try changing how you hold the client, altering the height of your couch or adjusting the position of your client on the couch or chair.

- If you are still having difficulty after trying various ways to apply STR, stop using that particular stretch.

Closing Remarks

In this chapter we have looked at the advantages and disadvantages of using different types of locks and have considered how and when to use massage tools. The section on commonly asked questions and troubleshooting tips, plus information concerning safety issues and how to measure the effectiveness of STR has helped provide the foundation for using this technique. Now you are ready to practice the three different forms of STR.

Quick Questions

1. Give an example of when you might use your palm to lock tissues.
2. Give examples of three kinds of clients for whom STR is not appropriate.
3. List the three types of STR.
4. For how long do you hold a lock at the end of a stretch?
5. List three ways you could measure the effectiveness of STR.

Soft Tissue Release Techniques

In this part of the book, you will find information on how to apply each of the three types of STR: passive, active-assisted and active. Each of the three chapters in part II follows the same format: First is a seven-step description of how to perform the technique. Next, key holds, moves and stances are described, using plenty of examples involving different muscles. This section provides condensed instructions and one representative photo for each technique, with page references to the complete instructions in chapters 6 to 8. To get a good understanding of the differences in application, you might want to flip back and forth among chapters 3, 4 and 5, comparing the photographs that are provided as overviews of the techniques. As you are aware, it is important to safeguard yourself and your clients when working, and each chapter therefore contains useful safety guidelines specific to the type of STR being described.

When performing STR, remember that some muscles are not usually shortened during the application. This is because it would be technically difficult to lock them once they have been placed in a shortened position. The table on page 26 lists those muscles that are usually shortened and those that are not.

At the end of each chapter, you will find a table indicating when each particular technique might be useful. These tables are not exhaustive, and with practice you will find that you are able to annotate them with notes from your own experience. Reading through these chapters will provide you with a clear understanding of the differences among the three different types of STR. You will then be ready to practice their application on different parts of the body as described in chapters 6 to 8.

Shortening of Muscles in Soft Tissue Release

Body area	Muscles
MUSCLES THAT ARE USUALLY SHORTENED	
Trunk	Rhomboids Pectorals
Lower limb	Hamstrings Iliacus Quadriceps Tibialis anterior Peroneals
Upper Limb	Triceps Biceps Wrist extensors Wrist flexors
MUSCLES THAT ARE *NOT* USUALLY SHORTENED	
Trunk	Upper trapezius Scalenes Levator scapulae Erector spinae
Lower limb	Plantar fascia of the foot Calf muscles Gluteals

Passive Soft Tissue Release

In this chapter you will discover how to perform passive STR by working through seven simple steps. To get you started with this form of the technique, there is a brief description of the key holds, moves and stances used for treating eight different muscles, along with safety guidelines and a chart illustrating when passive STR may be indicated. Reading this chapter and answering the Quick Questions will give you a good understanding of how passive STR is applied.

Introduction to Passive Soft Tissue Release

Passive soft tissue release is an excellent method of stretching that may be used as a stand-alone technique through clothing or incorporated into a holistic massage. In this form of STR, the therapist shortens a muscle, locks it and then stretches it. The client remains passive throughout but of course may provide feedback regarding the intensity of the stretch.

How to Do Passive STR

To perform passive STR, follow these steps:

1. Identify the muscle to be stretched and the direction of the muscle fibres.
2. Ensure the muscle is in a neutral position. Neutral means that the muscle is neither shortened too much nor stretched. Usually, this requires the therapist to passively shorten the muscle (the planter fascia and calf are exceptions to this rule).

   Some muscles (especially hamstrings) are prone to cramp when shortened. The likelihood of cramping increases after exercise. It is therefore sometimes a good idea to incorporate STR with oil massage, thus aiding the relaxation of muscle fibres before shortening the muscle and decreasing the likelihood of cramping when these muscles are shortened.

3. Explain the procedure to the client. Tell the client that *you* will be performing the stretch, and all he or she needs to do is relax. The muscle on which you are working should be relaxed.

   Gently shaking a limb encourages muscle relaxation and is useful when working with clients who find it difficult to 'switch off' and relax.

4. Whilst keeping the muscle in the neutral position, gently lock the muscle to fix the fibres. (See chapter 2 for a variety of locking methods.) Start proximally, nearest to the origin of the muscle.

TIP Generally, the origin of the muscle is that part closest to the midline of the body and least movable. Usually, when a muscle contracts, the insertion moves closer to the origin.

5. Whilst maintaining your lock, stretch the muscle. This will mean moving the body part in such a way that the muscle goes from a shortened to a lengthened position. For example, if you needed to flex a joint to shorten the muscle, you will need to extend the joint to stretch it.

6. Once the muscle has been stretched, release your lock and return the muscle to neutral.

7. Choose another point to fix the muscle, working proximally to distally. Repeat steps 4 to 6 until you reach the distal tendons of the muscle.

   To really focus your stretch on a particular area, place your locks close together, perhaps a centimetre apart, as you work from proximal to distal on a muscle. For a more general, less localized stretch, place your locks 3 to 4 centimetres apart.

Get feedback from your client. Some clients do not feel much of a stretch, simply the pressure of the lock. If you are applying the technique correctly, the stretch will increase as you work on the more distal aspects of the muscle. Stop if the client reports pain.

When applying STR, always work proximally to distally. This has the effect of making the stretch more and more intense. If you start distally, the stretch will already be intense. It is possible to perform STR on most muscles by working proximally to distally. However, when working muscles such as the rhomboids and pectoralis major, you may find that the area in which you need to lock is much smaller, and so you cannot follow this rule quite so easily.

Incorporating STR With Oil Massage

You can see that it would be easy to incorporate STR with oil massage. After the application of oil, put a thin towel over the area and apply STR through the towel. Be aware that working this way provides a much stronger lock than working through clothing or on bare skin because the fronds of the towel grip the oil. In fact, it is much easier to apply STR this way than on bare skin or through clothing. Remove the towel, clear the area with more massage and repeat. You will discover that if you do this three times (i.e., massage, STR; massage, STR; massage, STR), on your third application of STR, your client will sense less of a stretch (and you will sense less resistance in tissues) because the soft tissues will have lengthened after your first two applications.

Key Holds, Moves and Stances for Passive STR

Illustrated here are eight areas of the body that lend themselves to passive STR: the calf, hamstrings, rhomboids, triceps, biceps, wrist and finger flexors and extensors and pectorals. You can find detailed instructions for these stretches in chapters 6 to 8, where you can compare them to the instructions for active-assisted and active techniques.

Calf

Stand at the end of the couch with your client in prone. Lock the client's calf using reinforced thumbs, just distal to the knee joint, perhaps in the centre of the calf. Each time you lock the fibres in this stretch, direct your pressure towards the knee rather than perpendicularly. Whilst maintaining your lock, use your thigh to dorsiflex the client's ankle.

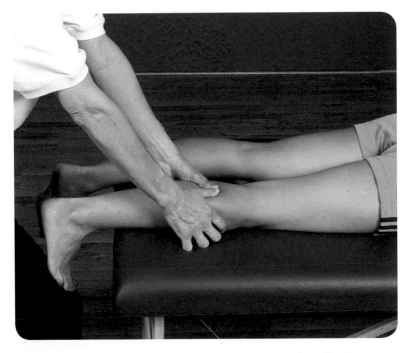

➤ See pages 88 to 92 for complete instructions for this stretch and a discussion of using reinforced thumbs.

Hamstrings

With your client in prone, passively shorten the hamstring muscles by flexing the client's knee. Lock the muscle close to the origin at the ischium. Each time you lock the fibres in this stretch, direct your pressure towards the ischium rather than perpendicularly. Whilst maintaining your lock, gently stretch the muscle by extending the knee.

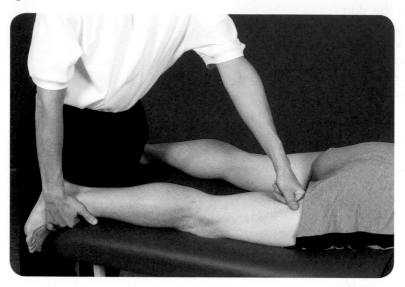

➤ See pages 81 to 83 for complete instructions for this stretch.

Rhomboids Prone

There are two methods of applying STR to rhomboids: The first is with your client prone on a treatment couch, and the second is with your client seated.

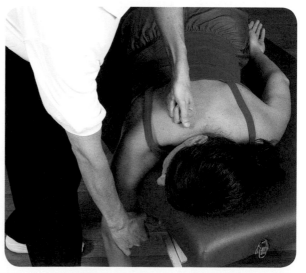

To treat the client in prone, position your client in prone on a treatment couch so she is able to flex at the shoulder. Whilst holding the client's arm to keep the rhomboids passively shortened, gently lock them, directing your pressure towards the spine. Maintain your lock and gently lower her arm into flexion so that the scapula protracts around the rib cage, stretching the rhomboids.

➤ See pages 65 to 67 for complete instructions for this stretch.

Rhomboids Sitting

With your client comfortably seated, gently hold her arm to passively retract the scapula, which shortens the rhomboids. Take up the slack in the skin, directing your pressure towards the spine. Whilst maintaining your lock, take the arm into flexion, passively protracting the scapula.

➤ See page 68 for complete instructions for this stretch.

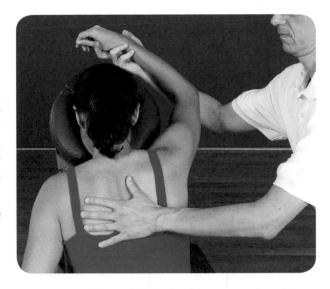

Triceps

Position your client in prone and make sure she is able to flex her arm at the elbow. Passively extend your client's elbow to shorten the muscle. Place your lock close to the origin, directing your pressure towards the shoulder. Whilst maintaining your lock, gently flex the elbow.

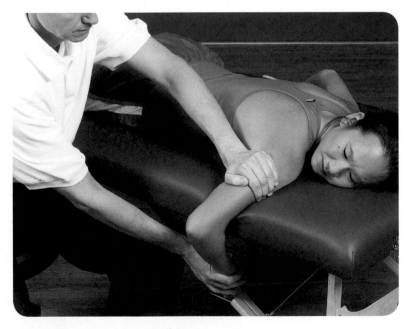

➤ See pages 114 to 115 for complete instructions for this stretch.

Biceps Brachii

With your client in supine and his elbow passively flexed, lock in gently to the biceps brachii, taking up slack in the skin as you direct pressure towards the armpit. Gently extend the elbow whilst maintaining your lock.

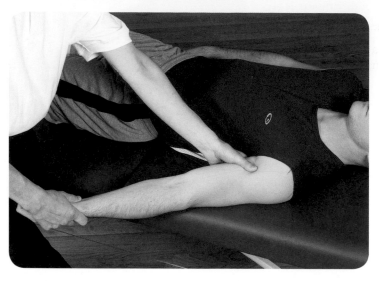

➤ See page 118 for complete instructions for this stretch.

Wrist and Finger Extensors

Gently extend your client's wrist. Lock into the bellies of the extensors on the lateral aspect of the forearm. Whilst maintaining your lock, gently flex the wrist.

➤ See page 120 for complete instructions for this stretch.

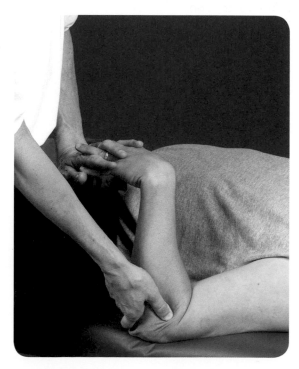

Wrist and Finger Flexors

Ask your client to flex her wrist. Gently lock into the common flexor origin. Gently extend the client's wrist whilst maintaining your lock.

➤ See page 123 for complete instructions for this stretch.

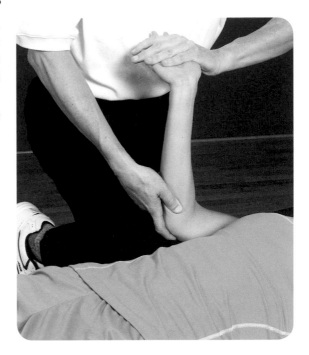

Pectorals

With your client in supine, take his arm into horizontal flexion and fix the tissues with a soft fist, directing your pressure towards the sternum rather than into the underlying ribs. Whilst maintaining your lock, gently take your client's arm from horizontal flexion into a more neutral position.

➤ See pages 69 to 70 for complete instructions for this stretch.

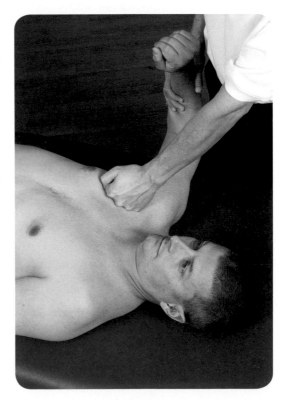

Safety Guidelines for Passive STR

Passive STR is safe and effective. However, it is useful to be aware of certain cautions before practicing this technique.

- When applying STR to the calf with your client in prone, make sure there are no locking clips on your treatment couch that may injure the dorsal surface of your client's foot during dorsiflexion. When working with your client in prone to apply STR to the calf or hamstrings, avoid pressing into the popliteal space at the back of the knee.

- When working rhomboids in prone, be careful not to place your client's entire body to the side of the treatment couch. It is safer and more stable to have your client lie diagonally across the couch.

- Whilst working the biceps brachii, avoid putting pressure into the anterior of the elbow, the cubital fossa.

- When applying STR, protect your thumbs. If you find your client does not experience a sensation of stretch and needs a firmer lock, use an alternate lock. If you find that using a different lock places stress on your own body, consider using active-assisted STR, which often enables you to apply greater pressure and alter your stance to a safer working position.

- When integrating STR with oil massage, remember that it is much easier to provide a lock when working through a towel than when working through clothing or on dry skin. For this reason, apply your locks cautiously until you gain feedback from the client as to the appropriateness of your pressure.

- When using passive STR, always get feedback from your client and stop if the client reports pain.

- When applying passive STR, all the usual massage contraindications apply. For example, do not apply STR to areas where there are varicose veins, broken skin, recent injuries or decreased sensitivity.

When Is Passive STR Indicated?

Passive STR may be used directly through clothing all over the body as part of a general stretching routine, or it may be incorporated into a holistic massage treatment. It is useful when used briskly before exercise with the aim of increasing joint range and overcoming cramps. It is used after exercise to help realign muscle fibres and overcome cramps. However, in both pre- and post-exercise settings, it should not be applied too deeply. It is also a useful tool for assessing muscle pliability.

Table 3.1 provides suggestions for when treatment for particular muscles can be useful.

Table 3.1 Situations in Which Passive STR Can Help

Muscle	Situation
Calf	■ To treat calf muscle cramps ■ For clients with tight calves ■ For clients engaged in physical activity involving the lower limbs, such as running, tennis or basketball ■ To treat clients who have been standing or walking for long periods ■ To increase range of motion at the ankle or knee ■ To treat clients who require increased ankle dorsiflexion (e.g., clients previously bedridden now required to stand) ■ To stretch out the calf muscles of clients who wear high-heeled footwear (which results in excessive plantar flexion and possible shortening of these muscles)
Hamstrings	■ For clients with tight hamstrings ■ For clients who sit for long periods, such as drivers or typists ■ For clients engaged in physical activity involving the lower limbs, such as running or basketball ■ To increase range of motion at the knee ■ For clients with excessive lumbar lordosis
Rhomboids	■ For clients who are engaged in physical activity involving the upper limbs, such as swimming, racket sports or rowing
Triceps	■ For clients whose physical activities involve prolonged or repetitive extension of the elbow, such as in racquet sports ■ For massage therapists ■ For treatment after immobilization of the elbow or shoulder ■ To increase elbow flexion
Biceps brachii	■ For clients whose physical activities involve prolonged or repetitive elbow flexion, such as rowing, digging or carrying ■ For treatment after immobilization of the elbow or shoulder ■ To increase range of movement at the elbow, particularly elbow extension
Wrist and finger extensors and flexors	■ For musicians such as guitarists, pianists, flautists or trumpet players ■ In the treatment of lateral epicondylitis (extensors) ■ In the treatment of medial epicondylitis (flexors) ■ For clients who perform repeated or prolonged flexion, such as typists, drivers or people carrying heavy bags ■ For clients whose sport requires gripping, such as in rock climbing or rowing ■ For massage therapists ■ For treatment after immobilization of the wrist or elbow
Pectorals	■ For clients with kyphotic postures ■ For clients who sit for long periods of time, such as drivers or typists ■ For bodybuilders, who may develop excessively tight pectorals relative to posterior trunk muscles ■ For clients who use the pectoralis major as part of their job, hobby or sport, such as trumpet players, tennis players or golfers

Quick Questions

1. What does it mean to say that a muscle is in a neutral position?
2. In passive STR, who performs the stretch, the client or the therapist?
3. Is a lock maintained whilst the muscle is being stretched?
4. Where is the client most likely to feel the stretch, at the proximal or distal end of the muscle?
5. Why should you be cautious when first integrating passive STR with oil massage?

Active-Assisted Soft Tissue Release

Use this chapter to get to grips with how to perform active-assisted STR. Start by reading through the seven simple steps and then try out the key holds, moves and stances used with this form of STR. This overview of using this technique on 15 muscles should help get you started. There are also safety guidelines and a chart illustrating when active-assisted STR may be indicated. Test whether you have understood the principles by attempting the Quick Questions at the end of the chapter.

Introduction to Active-Assisted Soft Tissue Release

Unlike passive STR (where tissues are shortened and locked by the therapist) or active STR (where the client does the techniques on himself or herself), active-assisted STR combines the efforts of both client and therapist. It is useful for working with clients who find it difficult to relax during treatment and also for those who like to be engaged with their treatment. It also enables the practitioner to apply more pressure when locking tissues, so it is useful for treating clients who do not feel the stretch of passive STR. The technique enables the therapist to use both hands if necessary to apply a firmer lock, which is helpful when treating large, bulky muscles such as hamstrings and quadriceps. Being able to reinforce a lock also enables the therapist to safeguard his or her wrists, fingers and thumbs.

Active-assisted STR is particularly useful as part of the rehabilitation process after joint immobilization. Not only does it increase range of motion in the joint, but it also improves strength in the associated muscles. It is a valuable rehabilitation technique because clients are encouraged to work within their pain-free range; after surgery, it may be a safer method of application than passive STR. With permission from medical personnel, it may be used early in the rehabilitation process to help keep joints lubricated and encourage a better alignment of collagen fibres than might otherwise occur if the joint were left immobile.

The biggest difference between active-assisted and passive STR is that in passive STR, the therapist is stretching a relaxed muscle. In active-assisted STR, the muscle being stretched is often contracting eccentrically as the client uses it to move the associated joint. With one or two exceptions, another difference is that the muscle being treated tends to be shortened in active-assisted STR instead of being in a neutral position.

How to Do Active-Assisted STR

To perform active-assisted STR, follow these steps:

1. Identify the muscle to be stretched and the direction of the fibres.

2. Ensure the muscle is in a neutral or shortened position. Neutral means that the muscle is neither shortened too much nor stretched. Neutral positions are used when treating the calf, foot, upper fibres of the trapezius, scalenes, levator scapulae and erector spinae muscles. When a muscle needs to be shortened—as with the hamstrings, iliacus, tibialis anterior, peroneals, quadriceps and pectorals—this shortening is performed by the client actively contracting the muscle in question. This is the position you need your client to hold when you lock the tissues.

3. Explain the procedure to the client. Demonstrate the movement you want your client to perform once you have locked the tissues. If, for example, you want to shorten the hamstrings, you could simply say, 'Please bend your knee', and most clients would understand this instruction. However, when treating peroneals and wrist flexors and extensors, for example, you need to be much more specific and demonstrate the action you want the client to perform. Many clients would not understand the command to evert the foot (needed for treating peroneals) and would need to be shown what to do when asked to flex or extend the wrist.

4. In the neutral or contracted position, lock the muscle to fix the fibres. Start proximally, nearest to the origin of the muscle.

5. Whilst maintaining your lock, ask your client to move in such a way that he or she feels a stretch in the muscle. How the client moves will vary depending on which muscle you are working. (See chapters 6 to 8 for photographs and descriptions of the movements for each muscle.)

6. Once the muscle has been stretched, release your lock and either let the muscle return to neutral or ask your client to contract the muscle again.

7. Choose another point to fix the muscle, working proximally to distally until you reach the distal tendons of the muscle.

Anatomy Reminder

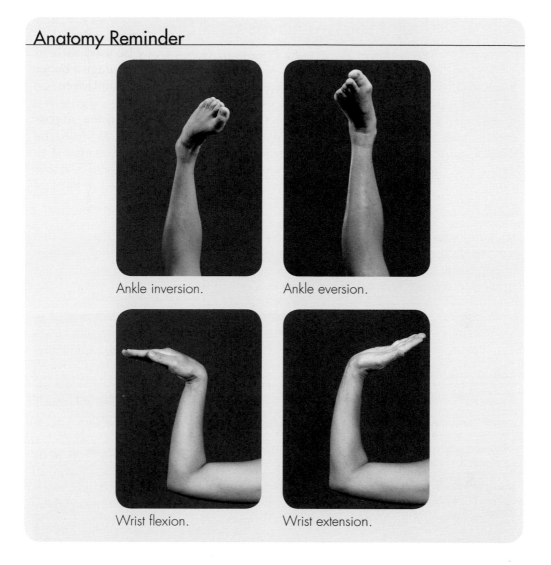

Ankle inversion.   Ankle eversion.

Wrist flexion.   Wrist extension.

Selecting Passive or Active-Assisted STR

When treating clients, avoid swopping between passive STR and active STR initially. If you use both methods, you may find that clients get confused and forget whether they are supposed to be taking part in the stretch. However, many clients soon learn what it is they are required to do for active-assisted STR, especially if they are receiving regular treatment from you. In subsequent treatments, you may find that you instinctively know which form of STR works best for which client; this is likely to vary depending on which muscle you are treating.

Remember that some clients never want to be actively engaged in their treatment, so active-assisted STR will never be appropriate, even in situations when you would view it as being beneficial. Some clients will always prefer the technique to be applied passively.

Key Holds, Moves and Stances
for Active-Assisted STR

Illustrated here are 15 areas of the body that lend themselves to active-assisted STR: the calf, foot, hamstrings, iliacus, tibialis anterior, peroneals, gluteals and quadriceps of the lower limbs; the upper trapezius, scalenes, levator scapulae, erector spinae and pectorals of the trunk; and the wrist and finger extensors and flexors. You can find detailed instructions for these stretches in chapters 6 to 8, where you can compare them to the passive and active techniques.

Calf

Lock the calf muscle just inferior to the knee joint, taking care not to press into the popliteal space at the back of the knee. Whilst maintaining your lock, ask your client to pull up her toes, thus dorsiflexing her foot and ankle. Once the client has done this, remove your lock and move to a new position.

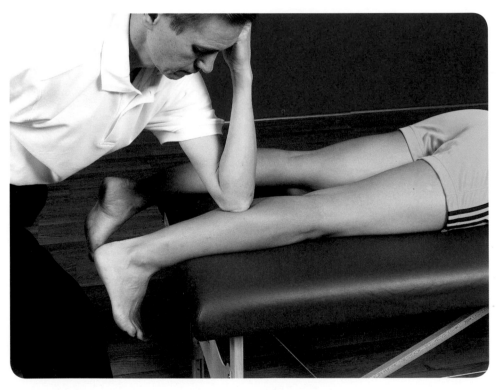

➤ See pages 93 to 94 for complete instructions for this stretch.

Foot

Position your client with his feet off the couch as shown; with the ankle in a neutral position, apply a gentle lock using a massage tool. Ask your client to pull up his toes, thus dorsiflexing the ankle and extending the toes. Work over the sole of each foot for a few minutes only.

➤ See pages 96 to 97 for complete instructions for this stretch.

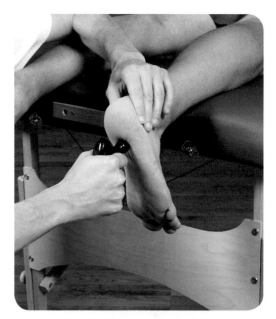

Hamstrings

Whilst your client is in a prone position, ask him to flex his knee. Using your elbow, lock the hamstrings close to the ischium. Direct your pressure towards the buttock to take up some of the slack in soft tissues before the stretch. Whilst maintaining your lock, ask your client to lower his leg back to the couch. Release your lock and ask the client to flex his knee again.

➤ See pages 84 to 85 for complete instructions for this stretch.

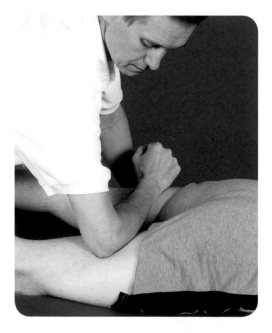

Iliacus

With your client positioned in side lying, hip flexed, lock into the iliacus (on the anterior surface of the ileum). Whilst maintaining your lock, ask your client to straighten his leg and extend his hip.

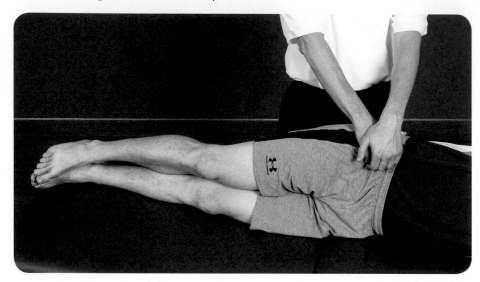

➤ See pages 110 to 111 for complete instructions for this stretch.

Tibialis Anterior

Whilst your client's ankle is in dorsiflexion, lock the tibialis anterior muscle using, for example, your elbow. Maintain your lock and ask your client to point her toes. Then release your lock and choose a new position, slightly more distal, for your second lock.

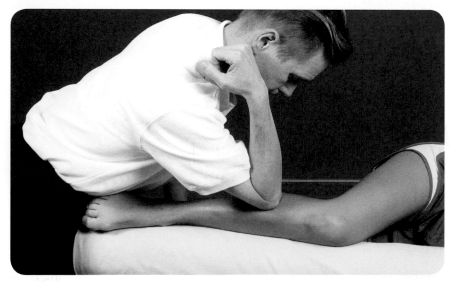

➤ See pages 104 to 105 for complete instructions for this stretch.

Peroneals

With your client positioned in side lying, ask her to evert her foot. Lock the muscle, which is now in a shortened position. Whilst maintaining your lock, ask the client to invert her foot. Work in a single line down the muscle, from proximal to distal, so that the client feels the stretch and it remains comfortable.

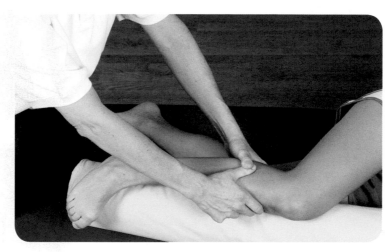

➤ See pages 106 to 107 for complete instructions for this stretch.

Gluteals

With your client in side lying, hip in neutral, use your forearm close to the elbow to lock the gluteals, directing your pressure towards the sacrum. Whilst maintaining your lock, ask your client to flex his hip. Repeat this for a few minutes, working on the area that feels most beneficial for the client.

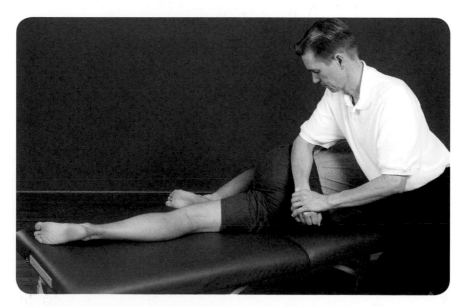

➤ See pages 108 to 109 for complete instructions for this stretch.

Quadriceps

With your client sitting, ask her to straighten her leg, which extends the knee. Once the muscle is actively shortened in this way, lock the quadriceps. Whilst maintaining your lock, ask your client to flex her knee. Once the knee is flexed, release your lock and repeat, placing a new lock slightly more distal to the first. Work your way down the quadriceps from hip to knee.

➤ See pages 100 to 101 for complete instructions for this stretch.

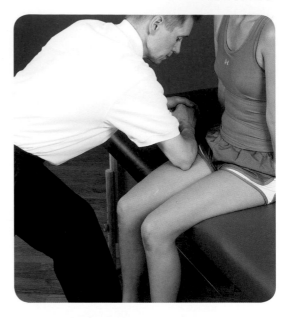

Upper Trapezius

With your client sitting, lock the upper fibres of the trapezius. Whilst maintaining your lock, ask your client to flex her neck laterally until she feels a comfortable stretch. Repeat three times and then repeat on the opposite side of the body.

➤ See page 74 for complete instructions for this stretch.

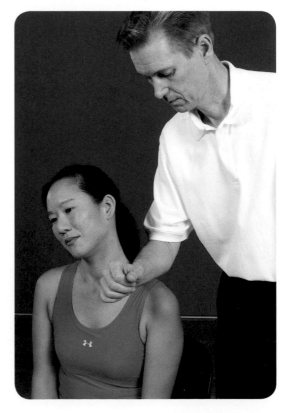

Scalenes

With your client sitting, gently lock the scalenes using your fingers. Ask your client to rotate her head away from you until she feels a comfortable stretch in the tissues. Repeat three times on both the left and right sides.

➤ See page 76 for complete instructions for this stretch.

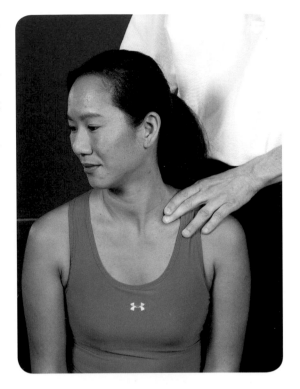

Levator Scapulae

Locate and lock the levator scapula. Whilst maintaining your lock, ask your client to rotate his head to about 45 degrees and then lower his chin to look to the floor. Ask your client to repeat this stretch three times; then use the same stretch on the opposite side of the body.

➤ See pages 72 to 73 for complete instructions for this stretch.

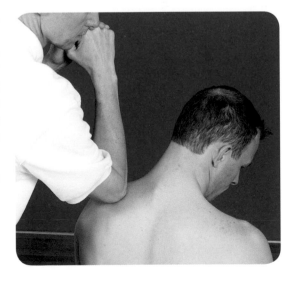

Erector Spinae (Spinalis)

With your client sitting, lock the tissues in the mid-thoracic area. Whilst maintaining your lock, ask your client to flex his neck. Release and repeat, placing your lock slightly superior to the first one.

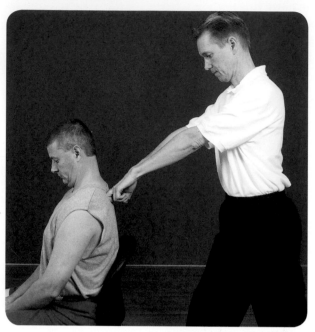

➤ See page 75 for complete instructions for this stretch.

Pectorals

Ask your client to take his arm across his body, actively shortening the pectoralis major. Using soft fists, lock the muscle, directing your pressure towards the sternum. Whilst maintaining your lock, ask your client to move his arm so that he feels a stretch in the pectorals.

➤ See page 71 for complete instructions for this stretch.

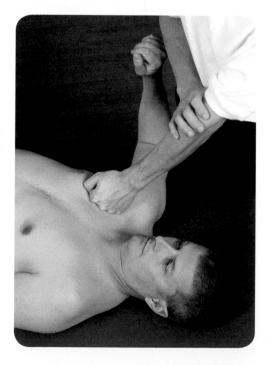

Wrist and Finger Extensors

Locate the bellies of the wrist and finger extensors by asking your client to extend his wrist. Lock the tissues. Whilst maintaining your lock, ask your client to flex his wrist. Repeat over the lateral aspect of the elbow where the muscle bellies are located.

➤ See page 121 for complete instructions for this stretch.

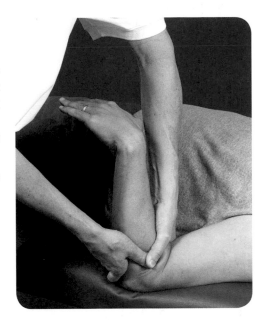

Wrist and Finger Flexors

Identify the muscles by asking the client to flex her wrist. Lock the tissues over the muscle bellies. Whilst maintaining your lock, ask your client to extend her wrist. Repeat this lock, stretch, lock, stretch sequence over the muscle bellies.

➤ See page 124 for complete instructions for this stretch.

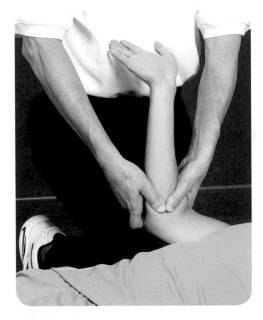

Safety Guidelines for Active-Assisted STR

The following guidelines will help keep active-assisted STR safe for you and your clients:

- Your usual massage contraindications apply. For example, do not use active-assisted STR if your client has varicose veins.

- When treating the calf and hamstring muscles, avoid pressing into the popliteal space behind the knee.

- When working, be aware of your posture and guard your back. For example, avoid unsupported spinal flexion when treating the calf.

- When working with a client with an injury to the tibialis anterior, avoid active-assisted STR to the calf. In this case, constant dorsiflexion will fatigue the tibialis anterior. An exception to this may be when a client has a dropped foot due to weakness in the tibialis anterior; in this case, active-assisted STR to the calf may actually be beneficial as part of a programme to increase strength in the ankle dorsiflexors.

- When working along the tibia and fibula, ensure that the client's knee is fully supported if he or she is positioned in side lying. If you are applying your elbows to access these strap-like muscles, work cautiously to avoid bruising the tissues against the underlying bones.

- When stretching the quadriceps of clients with anterior knee pain, recognize you may not be able to work to as distal a point as usual. This is because the closer to the knee you place your lock, the greater the stretch and the greater the pressure on the patella. Whilst this may be beneficial in the long term in overcoming patellofemoral pain due to tight quadriceps, it could be painful during the stretch itself.

- When working the scalenes, take care not to press too deeply. Be sure to get feedback from the client.

When Is Active-Assisted STR Indicated?

Overall, active-assisted STR is useful in these situations:

- When working with clients who find it difficult to relax during treatment
- When treating clients who like to be engaged with their treatment
- When it is necessary to apply more pressure to lock tissues
- When treating clients who do not feel the stretch of passive STR
- When treating large, bulky muscles such as hamstrings and quadriceps
- When it is essential for you to safeguard your wrists, fingers and thumbs
- When muscle strengthening is required, perhaps after immobilization of a joint

Table 4.1 provides suggestions for when active-assisted treatment to particular muscles may be useful.

Table 4.1 Situations in Which Active-Assisted STR Can Help

Muscle	Situation
Calf	■ For clients with tight calves ■ For clients engaged in physical activity involving the lower limbs, such as running, tennis or basketball ■ To treat clients who have been standing or walking for long periods ■ To increase range of motion at the ankle or knee ■ To treat clients who require increased ankle dorsiflexion (e.g., clients previously bedridden now required to stand) ■ To stretch out the calf muscles of clients who wear high-heeled footwear (which results in excessive plantar flexion and possible shortening of these muscles) ■ For use as part of a programme to help strengthen the tibialis anterior
Foot	■ For clients with plantar fasciitis ■ For clients with Achilles tendon problems
Hamstrings	■ For clients with tight hamstrings ■ For clients who sit for long periods, such as drivers or typists ■ For clients engaged in physical activity involving the lower limbs, such as cycling, running or basketball ■ To increase range of motion at the knee ■ For clients with excessive lumbar lordosis ■ With medical permission, after knee surgery or immobilization of the knee
Iliacus	■ For clients with tight hip flexors ■ For clients engaged in physical activity that requires repetitive or prolonged hip flexion, such as running, rowing, cycling or jockeying ■ For clients who sit for long periods, such as drivers ■ To increase hip extension ■ For clients engaged in riding motorcycles for long periods
Tibialis anterior	■ For clients with tight tibialis anterior muscles ■ For clients engaged in sporting activities that require repeated or prolonged dorsiflexion, such as running or tennis ■ After walking uphill for long periods ■ After standing for long periods ■ To help increase plantar flexion, should that be required, after ankle joint immobilization
Peroneals	■ For clients with tight peroneals, often those with 'flat feet' ■ To help increase inversion after immobilization of the ankle joint ■ For clients engaged in physical activity that uses the leg muscles ■ For clients who are prone to repetitive eversion of the ankle, such as horse riders
Gluteals	■ For clients engaged in physical activity that requires repetitive or prolonged hip extension or abduction, such as running, jumping or ice skating

(continued)

Table 4.1 *(continued)*

Muscle	Situation
Quadriceps	■ For clients with tight quadriceps ■ For clients engaged in physical activity involving the lower limbs, such as cycling, running or jumping ■ To increase range of motion at the knee ■ To increase knee flexion
Upper trapezius, scalenes, levator scapulae, erector spinae (spinalis)	■ For clients with tight neck muscles ■ For clients who spend long periods sitting, such as writers, drivers or typists ■ For singers ■ To increase range of motion in the neck ■ For treatment after immobilization of the neck ■ During seated chair massage routines by therapists working in this capacity ■ For clients who suffer headaches induced by increased muscle tension ■ For clients needing treatment after immobilization of the scapula or as part of the rehabilitation process after injury to the shoulder, especially for the upper trapezius and levator scapulae ■ For anyone who performs repetitive or prolonged shoulder activities, especially those involving overarm movements, such as tennis, swimming or overarm bowling ■ For clients who hold static postures for prolonged periods, such as painters, artists or models
Pectorals	■ For clients with tight pectorals ■ For clients who have kyphotic postures ■ To increase horizontal extension at the shoulder ■ For treatment after immobilization of the shoulder joint (when the client has been in a sling, for example) ■ For clients who perform repeated or prolonged movements of the shoulder, especially those activities requiring adduction, forward flexion and horizontal flexion of the shoulder, such as rock climbing, racquet sports or swimming ■ For clients who maintain prolonged forward flexion at the shoulder, such as cyclists or drivers
Wrist and finger extensors and flexors	■ For musicians whose performance requires repeated finger movements, such as guitarists, pianists, flautists or trumpet players ■ In the treatment of lateral epicondylitis (extensors) ■ In the treatment of medial epicondylitis (flexors) ■ For clients who perform repeated or prolonged flexion, such as typists, drivers or people carrying heavy bags ■ For clients whose sport requires gripping, such as rock climbing or rowing ■ For massage therapists ■ For treatment after immobilization of the wrist or elbow

Quick Questions

1. Who performs the stretch in active-assisted STR, the client, the therapist or both?
2. For which sort of client might active-assisted STR be useful?
3. Why is this form of STR useful for rehabilitation after joint immobilization?
4. What is the biggest difference between passive and active-assisted STR?
5. Why should you avoid swopping between passive and active-assisted STR when working with a client for the first time?

Active Soft Tissue Release

Passive and active-assisted STR are techniques you would use as a therapist when treating clients. In this chapter, you will discover how to perform active STR, a technique you might use on yourself or teach to your clients to use as part of a home care programme. Included here are brief descriptions of the key holds, moves and stances used for treating eight muscles, with accompanying photographs, along with safety guidelines and a chart illustrating when active STR may be indicated. As with the previous two chapters, answering the Quick Questions will help establish your understanding of how active STR is applied.

Introduction to Active Soft Tissue Release

It is possible to perform active soft tissue release on many of the muscles in the body. To do this, you apply a lock to yourself and perform the stretch yourself, with no assistance from a therapist. Unlike passive soft tissue release, the muscle involved will be actively rather than passively shortened. This means you will lock into a contracted rather than a relaxed muscle. Nevertheless, the technique seems to be effective at releasing tension in the muscle and is useful as a quick fix when a therapist is unavailable.

How to Do Active STR

To perform active STR, follow these steps:

1. Identify the muscle to be stretched and the direction of the fibres.
2. Shorten the muscle. This means concentrically contracting it. How you do this will depend on which muscle you are working. If you are working your hamstrings, for example, flex your knee; if you are working your triceps,

extend your elbow. You do not need to fully contract the muscle. In fact, in some cases, this makes STR impossible. For example, if you fully flexed your elbow to contract your biceps, you would not be able to lock the muscle because you would have no space to grip it.

3. With the muscle gently shortened, lock the fibres. Start proximally, nearest the origin of the muscle.

4. Once the fibres are locked, actively lengthen the muscle. Maintain your lock throughout the movement.

5. Once the muscle is lengthened, remove your lock.

6. Shorten the muscle again.

7. Choose a new place to lock, slightly more distal to your first position. Repeat.

Stop when you reach the distal tendons of the muscle. If you have performed STR correctly, you should feel the stretch increase as you work from proximal to distal on the muscle.

TIP To be really good at performing STR, you need to know your muscles and the actions they bring about. If necessary, keep an anatomy text close at hand whilst working through this book.

Active STR as Part of a Home Care Programme

Active STR is a useful technique to share with clients as part of their home care programme. After all, if you are seeing a client once a week for treatment, the client still has another six days during which to manage the condition. Providing clients with tips on applying STR themselves may help address the underlying condition and keep the clients engaged with their own rehabilitation. In addition, many therapists find it useful to apply STR to their own forearms, which, despite good practice, often become excessively tight and develop trigger spots.

Key Holds, Moves and Stances for Active STR

Illustrated here are eight areas of the body that lend themselves to active STR: the plantar fascia on the sole of the foot, hamstrings, quadriceps, calf, wrist and finger extensors and flexors, biceps brachii and triceps. You can find detailed instructions for these stretches in chapters 6 to 8, where you can compare active STR to the passive and active-assisted techniques.

Foot

Sit down and place your foot on a tennis ball or spiky therapy ball with your ankle in neutral. Gently extend your toes, keeping your ankle in dorsiflexion. Work over the sole, moving the ball to discover which aspect of the fascia is tight and would benefit most from the stretch.

➤ See pages 98 to 99 for complete instructions for this stretch.

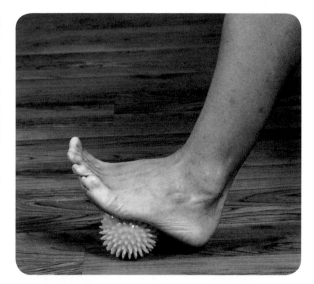

Hamstrings

Lie on your back, shorten the muscle by flexing your knee and place a tennis ball over part of your hamstring muscles. Whilst holding the tennis ball as shown, gently extend your knee. Place your first lock (using the ball) near the ischium and gradually work down towards your knee with subsequent locks.

➤ See pages 86 to 87 for complete instructions for this stretch.

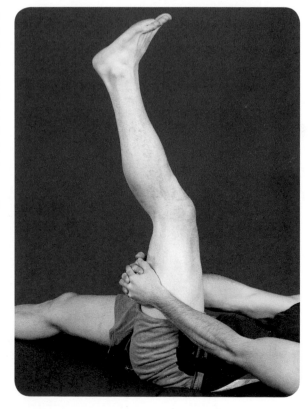

Quadriceps

Whilst resting face down, practice positioning the ball on various parts of your thigh; notice where you feel the most stretch. Position the ball first near your hip and work towards your knee with subsequent locks.

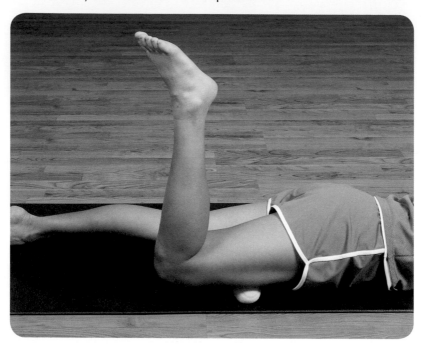

➤ See pages 102 to 103 for complete instructions for this stretch.

Calf

Place your calf on a ball as shown. Gently dorsiflex your ankle.

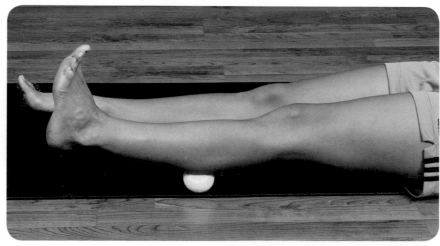

➤ See page 95 for complete instructions for this stretch.

Wrist and Finger Extensors

Locate the bellies of your wrist and finger extensor muscles. Gently lock into the tissues with your wrist in extension. Whilst maintaining your lock, gently flex your wrist. Work all over your wrist extensors from proximal (near the elbow) to distal (near the wrist).

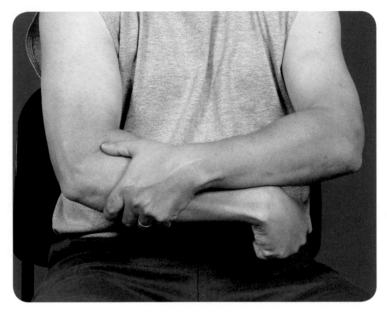

➤ See page 122 for complete instructions for this stretch.

Wrist and Finger Flexors

Identify the bellies of your wrist and finger flexors. With your wrist in flexion, gently lock into this area, pulling the tissues gently towards the elbow. Whilst maintaining your lock, gently extend your wrist. Work your way from elbow to wrist.

➤ See pages 125 to 126 for complete instructions for this stretch.

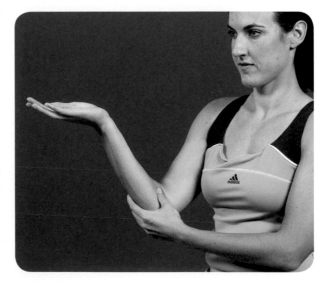

Biceps Brachii

With your arm in flexion, gently grip your biceps muscle. Gently extend your elbow whilst maintaining your grip.

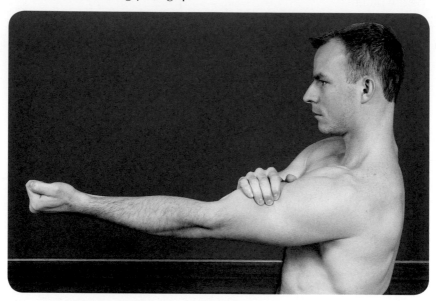

➤ See page 119 for complete instructions for this stretch.

Triceps

Extend your arm and grip your triceps muscle. Whilst maintaining your grip, gently flex your elbow.

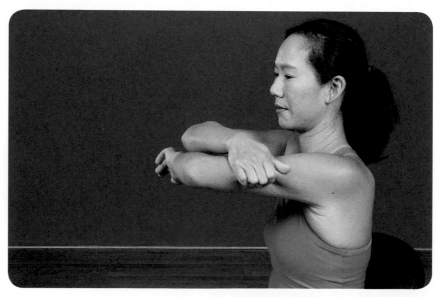

➤ See pages 116 to 117 for complete instructions for this stretch.

Safety Guidelines for Active STR

Active STR is safe and effective. However, it is useful to be aware of certain cautions before practicing this technique, especially because in some cases there may be quite a lot of pressure to body tissues.

- Avoid active STR if you have had a recent injury or if you bruise easily.
- Do not transfer your whole body weight onto the tennis or therapy ball when applying STR to the plantar fascia and never try to stand on the ball.
- If you are using STR to self-treat plantar fasciitis or golfer's or tennis elbow, proceed with caution: apply the technique gently for a maximum of three minutes. Most people will find active STR alleviates some of the discomfort of these conditions. However, if your condition seems aggravated within 12 hours of application, do not repeat STR. Avoid the use of active STR if you lack sensitivity in the area being treated.
- Be careful not to overwork any one area. Although soft tissue release is a great way to stretch muscles, stop after you have applied STR two or three times to one area. See how that area feels the next day. If it feels sore, do not repeat STR.
- Be careful when using STR to help lengthen the tissues acting on a joint that has been immobilized. Skin integrity may be compromised at this time. The skin may be particularly fragile if you have been in a plaster cast, for example.
- Avoid active deep STR before a sporting event. Whilst it may be tempting to use the technique to stretch out hamstrings before a race, for example, deep stretching should be avoided because it may decrease muscle power.
- Be careful when using your thumbs to lock into tissues, as in treating the wrist flexors and extensors. These muscles are relatively small, and little pressure is required to fix them during the stretch. If you discover that applying STR in this way starts to hurt your thumbs, have passive STR done for you or find an alternative method to lock the tissues.

When Is Active STR Indicated?

Active STR may be used directly through clothing all over the body as part of a general stretching routine. It is also useful for addressing trigger points: a ball or massage tool may be placed over the point and pressure applied before the stretch.

Table 5.1 provides suggestions for when active treatment to particular muscles may be useful.

Table 5.1   Situations in Which Active STR Can Help

Muscle	Situation
Plantar fascia	■ To treat plantar fasciitis ■ After standing for long periods ■ After exercise, such as running or walking ■ To treat foot muscle cramps ■ To help regain flexibility in the plantar fascia after an injury such as an ankle sprain ■ To help regain flexibility in foot muscles after immobilization in a cast, such as with a ruptured Achilles tendon
Hamstrings	■ To treat tight hamstrings ■ After sitting for long periods ■ To increase knee extension after immobilization of the knee joint
Quadriceps	■ After exercise involving the quadriceps, such as walking, running or stepping ■ After standing for long periods of time
Calf	■ After exercise that uses the calf muscles a lot, such as tennis, running or basketball ■ After immobilization of the ankle
Wrist and finger extensors and flexors	■ For typists ■ For tennis players (extensors), golfers (flexors) and drivers (flexors) ■ After carrying heavy bags ■ For sports that require gripping, such as rock climbing or rowing ■ For massage therapists ■ After immobilization of the wrist or elbow
Biceps brachii	■ For any activity with prolonged or repetitive elbow flexion, such as rowing, digging or carrying ■ After immobilization of the elbow or shoulder
Triceps	■ For any activity involving prolonged or repetitive extension of the elbow, such as tennis ■ For massage therapists ■ After immobilization of the elbow or shoulder

Quick Questions

1. How do I shorten the muscle I want to work on?
2. Do I contract first and then lock, or lock and then contract?
3. How do I know which way to work along the muscle?
4. Can I use STR if I bruise easily?
5. For how long can I apply active STR to one muscle?

Applying Soft Tissue Release

The three chapters in part III of *Soft Tissue Release* provide detailed information about how to apply STR to various muscles of the body. In chapter 6 you will learn how to apply STR to muscles of the trunk, including the rhomboids, pectorals, levator scapulae, the upper fibres of the trapezius, the erector spinae and the scalenes. Chapter 7 focuses on the lower limbs; you will learn the techniques to be used on the hamstrings, calf, foot, quadriceps, tibialis anterior, peroneals, gluteals and iliacus. Chapter 8 provides examples of how to apply STR to the muscles of the upper limbs, including stretches for the biceps, triceps and wrist and finger flexors and extensors.

Each chapter contains an overview chart detailing which forms of STR may be used for each muscle. Photographs showing start and end positions are provided along with step-by-step guidelines, plus the advantages and disadvantages of each stretch. There are plenty of helpful tips and even some Client Talk boxes, with examples of how some of the stretches have been used in real-life situations. As usual, there are Quick Questions with which to test yourself at the end of each chapter. Use these chapters in any order to help you master all three types of STR.

6

Soft Tissue Release for the Trunk

This chapter outlines how to apply soft tissue release to the trunk. Here you will find comparisons between applying passive, active-assisted and active STR to each of the major muscle groups of the trunk. Notice, however, that not all three versions of STR can be applied to all muscle groups (see table 6.1). In fact, active STR is rarely used in treating the trunk muscles listed here.

Table 6.1   Types of STR Used on Trunk Muscles

	TYPE OF STR		
Muscle	**Passive**	**Active-assisted**	**Active**
Rhomboids	✓	-	-
Pectorals	✓	✓	-
Levator scapulae	-	✓	-
Upper trapezius	-	✓	-
Erector spinae (spinalis)	-	✓	-
Scalenes	-	✓	-

- **Passive STR:** It is useful to apply STR passively to rhomboids and pectorals. However, when working with tissues of the neck, active-assisted STR is a more appropriate method of application. Active-assisted STR puts the client in charge of his or her own neck movements and therefore the degree of stretch received.

- **Active-assisted STR:** This technique is a useful method of safely stretching the pectorals, levator scapulae, upper trapezius, erector spinae and scalenes. It may be used on rhomboids, but with the client in prone, these muscles are quickly fatigued. Applying active-assisted STR to the rhomboids also makes it difficult for the therapist to firmly lock the tissues, which are relatively small and become shortened when concentrically contracted. For these reasons, illustrations of active-assisted STR to the rhomboids have not been included here.

■ **_Active STR:_** Whilst trunk muscles are often included in an overall stretching routine, these muscles are generally not stretched using active STR. This is because it is fairly difficult to lock the tissues correctly without causing strain to other body parts.

On the following pages are detailed instructions for applying passive, active-assisted or active STR to many of the muscles of the trunk, including tips that may help you apply these techniques.

Passive STR: Rhomboids Prone

Step 1: Position your client in prone on a treatment couch so she is able to flex at the shoulder. To do this you will need to position your client so that her arm can hang off the couch. A safe way to do this is to have her lie at an angle on the couch, feet positioned at the corner opposite to the arm you are working on. With your client in this position, shorten the rhomboids by passively retracting the scapula.

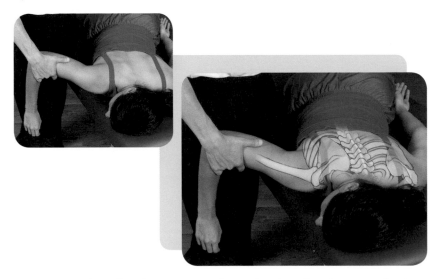

Step 2: Whilst holding the client's arm to keep the rhomboids passively shortened, gently lock them, directing your pressure towards the spine. As you can see from the skeleton illustration, the ribs curve outward. It is therefore important to direct your pressure towards the spine rather than perpendicularly because pressing into the ribs would be uncomfortable for the client.

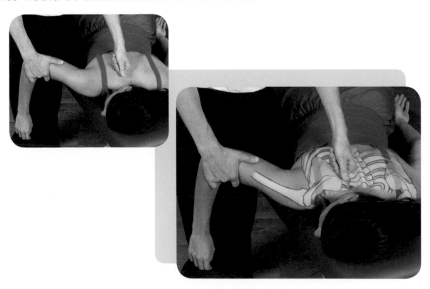

Step 3: Whilst maintaining your lock, gently lower your client's arm into flexion so that the scapula protracts around the rib cage, stretching the rhomboids.

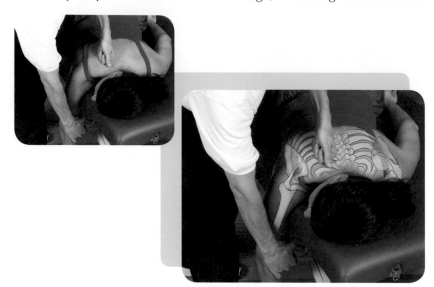

Relatively speaking, rhomboids are a small group of muscles and cannot be worked in lines as some other muscles can. Change the position of your lock to any point on the rhomboids as you repeat the procedure.

TIP You may need to practice repositioning your client to ensure flexion at the shoulder. If the client is not correctly positioned, this technique may cause pressure on the brachial plexus in the armpit, which could be uncomfortable.

If you find using your fist uncomfortable for your wrist, try using your forearm for the lock. Elbows should be used with caution over this bony area.

CLIENT TALK

I found active-assisted STR to the rhomboids in prone to be particularly useful when I was treating a female rower with large musculature. By combining this technique with lots of oil massage, I was able to get good leverage on the client's muscles and use my elbow to localize the stretch to specific areas of tightness. However, I did need to work through a facecloth because it was quite difficult to get a firm enough lock on the skin alone.

Advantage   You have considerable leverage and will be able to fix the muscles well.

Disadvantages   If the client is not correctly positioned, this technique may cause uncomfortable pressure on the brachial plexus in the armpit. ■ Be careful to use appropriate posture when lifting and lowering the client's arm. ■ This technique cannot easily be incorporated into an oil massage because it requires the client to be positioned diagonally on the treatment couch, which would mean moving the client several times during treatment. ■ With good leverage, some therapists accidentally press too hard; this is especially uncomfortable when working over ribs. ■ Unless your client is engaged in regular physical activity, it may be unlikely he or she needs the rhomboids stretched. Many clients have kyphotic postures, with protracted shoulders. When the shoulders are protracted, the rhomboids are lengthened. Do you need to stretch them further?

Passive STR: Rhomboids Sitting

Step 1: With your client comfortably seated, gently hold her arm to passively retract the scapula, shortening the rhomboids. Take up the slack in the skin, directing your pressure towards the spine.

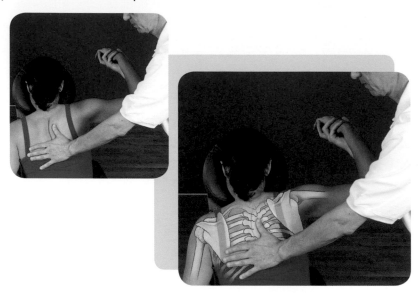

Step 2: Whilst maintaining your lock, take the arm into flexion, which passively protracts the scapula.

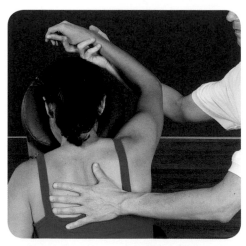

Advantage   In this position, you have less leverage and are therefore less likely to apply too much pressure. As a result, this is a good method of working with clients who are especially sensitive to pressure.

Disadvantages   Be careful to safeguard your thumbs. ■ It is difficult to perform passive STR on clients with long or heavy limbs. ■ Some clients find it hard to relax during passive STR and will always tense their limbs. ■ When the client is sitting, the muscles of the posterior trunk are not as relaxed as in prone.

Passive STR

Step 1: With your client in supine, take his arm into horizontal flexion and fix the tissues with a soft fist, directing your pressure towards the sternum rather than into the underlying ribs. You may want to explain to your client where you are going to position your fist for the lock because some clients may find this invasive.

TIP If you find it tricky to apply your lock, cushion the lock by working through a facecloth folded into fourths.

Step 2: Whilst maintaining your lock, gently take your client's arm from horizontal flexion into a more neutral position.

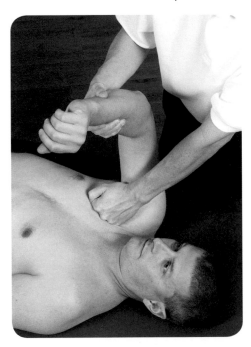 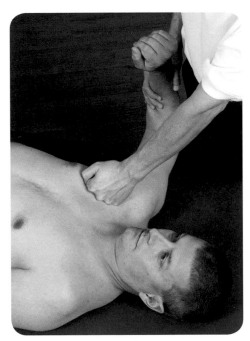

You can see from these photographs that the movement is small, requiring only a subtle change in arm position for the client to experience this stretch. When treating a female client, you will need to focus on the upper fibres of the pectoralis major and avoid working through breast tissue. When treating male clients, you may work over a greater part of the muscle.

TIP Avoid pressing downward into the ribs. If you find that your fists are too large for the small area on which you need to work, try using the pads of your fingers and gently reinforce one hand over the other.

Some clients do not feel the stretch immediately. This will require you to practice the technique by applying your pressure from various angles and stretching the tissues by moving the client's arm in varying degrees of abduction. However, clients with kyphotic postures may feel the stretch immediately because they have shortened pectorals.

Advantage   This technique is relatively easy to incorporate into a holistic massage treatment.

Disadvantages   It takes practice to direct pressure towards the sternum rather than downward into the ribs. ■ Your hands may be too large to use your fists, especially if the client has a small frame. In this case, use your fingers but exercise care because there will be an increased likelihood of pressing into the ribs. ■ It takes practice to know at which angle to abduct the arm, and the angle needed to facilitate the stretch varies considerably between clients. ■ This stretch cannot be applied easily to clients with large breasts. ■ It can be difficult finding the correct method of supporting the upper limb when working with larger clients. ■ Clients with large and well-developed pectorals are unlikely to feel passive STR to the pectorals; a considerably stronger lock is required to fix the tissues of these clients.

Active-Assisted STR

Step 1: Ask your client to move his arm across his body, which actively shortens the pectoralis major. Using soft fists, lock the muscle and direct your pressure towards the sternum.

Step 2: Whilst maintaining your lock, ask your client to move his arm so he can feel the stretch in his pectorals. The client will need to move his arm from horizontal flexion into a more neutral position.

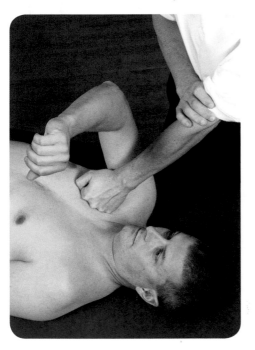 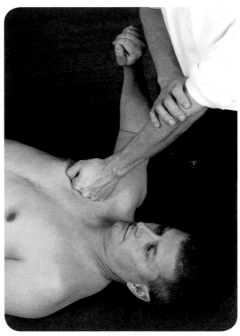

Step 3: Release and repeat steps 1 and 2 three times on each side of the body.

Advantages   The client will be able to locate the precise position where he or she feels the stretch. ▪ You can reinforce the lock using two soft fists or reinforced fingers.

Disadvantage   It can be tricky at first to find the best place to stand as the client moves his or her arm in search of the stretch. However, once the client finds the position, the treatment can proceed without disruption.

Applying STR to the levator scapulae and upper trapezius is particularly useful when treating clients with shoulder problems because these muscles both affect the scapula. These are safe stretches to use on the neck area because the stretch is performed actively, within the client's comfort level. It is therefore unlikely that the tissues would ever be overstretched. The technique may be used as part of an overall neck flexibility programme and to maintain length in these muscles, which are prone to increased tension.

Active-Assisted STR

Step 1: Locate the levator scapula.

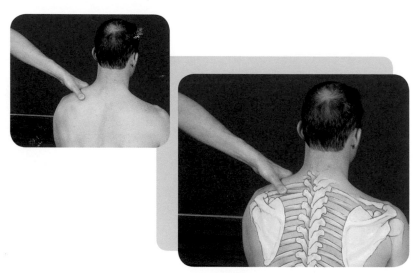

Step 2: Lock the muscle. This is a strap-like muscle and is often hypertonic (extremely tight).

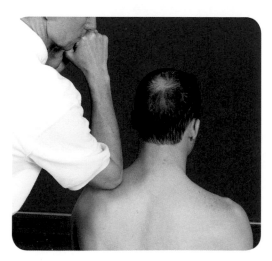

Step 3: Whilst maintaining your lock, ask your client to rotate his head to about 45 degrees and then lower his chin to look to the floor. Repeat three times and then apply the same stretch to the opposite side of the body.

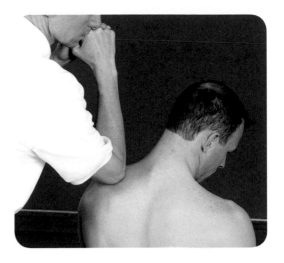

TIP This muscle is so hypertonic in many clients that they cannot tolerate a stretch at all; simply locking the muscle provides some relief for their tension.

CLIENT TALK

I taught two telephonists how to perform active-assisted STR. They used it gently in treating each other, taking turns throughout the day, in order to alleviate tension in each other's neck muscles.

Advantages   When you work in this position, you have easy access to the muscle and good leverage. ■ There is little danger that soft tissues of the neck will be overstretched because the client is in charge of the stretch. Provided that the client is reminded to stretch only within a comfortable, pain-free range, this technique should always be a safe way to use STR to stretch this muscle.

Disadvantages   This muscle is so hypertonic in many clients that they cannot tolerate a stretch. ■ For the stretch to be really effective, it is essential that the client be shown specifically where to move his or her head once the therapist has locked the tissues. ■ Make sure that for each new lock, the client's neck is in neutral, with the head facing forward.

Active-Assisted STR

Step 1: With your client sitting, lock the upper fibres of the trapezius.

Step 2: Whilst maintaining your lock, ask your client to laterally flex her neck as shown until she feels a comfortable stretch.

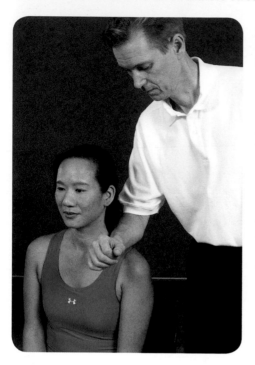 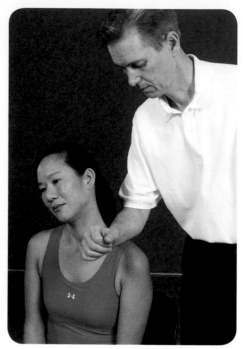

Step 3: Repeat three times and then repeat the same stretch on the opposite side of the body.

Advantages   When you work in this position, you have easy access to the muscle and good leverage. ▪ There is little danger that soft tissues of the neck will be overstretched because the client is in charge of the stretch. Provided that the client is reminded to stretch only within a comfortable, pain-free range, this technique should always be a safe way to use STR to stretch this muscle. ▪ With practice, and by working with the client, you will be able to alter the direction of pressure to localize the stretch to different fibres in the upper trapezius.

Disadvantage   Be careful not to press into bony structures, such as the clavicle and acromion process.

Active-Assisted STR

Step 1: With your client sitting, lock the tissues in the mid-thoracic area. In this photograph, the therapist has chosen to use his knuckles.

Step 2: Whilst maintaining your lock, ask your client to flex his neck.

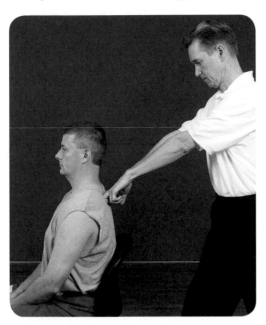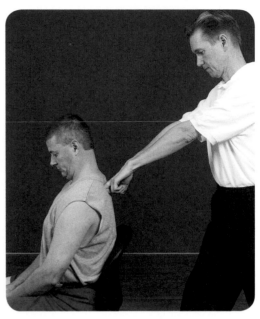

Step 3: Release and repeat, placing your lock slightly superior to the first one. Repeat as you work superiorly towards the neck. If you are performing STR correctly, your client will feel an increasing stretch as you move up the erector spinae.

Advantage   Clients usually find this to be a comfortable stretch. It can be performed with the client in a sitting position.

Disadvantages   It is difficult to get a good lock on these tissues. As shown, locking presses the client forward. It takes practice for the client to learn to remain upright, perhaps pressing back against your hands. ■ Be careful to avoid overuse of your fingers or thumbs.

Active-Assisted STR

Step 1: With your client sitting, gently lock the scalenes using your fingers.

Step 2: Ask your client to rotate her head away from you until she feels a comfortable stretch in the tissues.

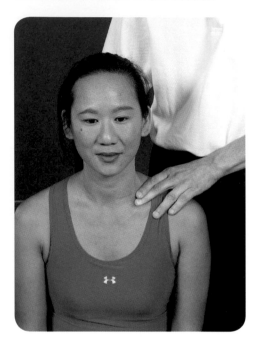 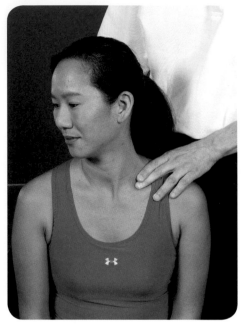

Step 3: Repeat the stretch three times on both the left and right sides.

Advantage   When you work in this position, there is little danger that soft tissues of the neck will be overstretched because the client is in charge of the stretch. Provided that the client is reminded to stretch only within a comfortable, pain-free range, this should always be a safe way to use STR to stretch this muscle.

Disadvantage   It takes practice to fix the scalenes while avoiding the vascular structures of the neck.

CLIENT TALK

I regularly applied active-assisted STR to the scalenes of a chauffeur who had complained of neck and shoulder pain associated with long-distance driving. The treatments tended to be fairly short and were combined with active stretches for the pectoral muscles, which the client was instructed to perform regularly whenever he had a break.

Quick Questions

1. When a therapist applies passive STR to rhomboids, why does the client need to have his or her arm positioned off the couch?

2. When applying active-assisted STR to pectorals, how might you dissipate the pressure of your lock?

3. Why is active-assisted STR to the levator scapulae a relatively safe method of stretching neck tissues?

4. When applying active-assisted STR to the upper fibres of the trapezius, which bony structures should you be aware of?

5. When active-assisted STR is applied to the erector spinae, does the client flex or extend once you have locked the tissues?

Soft Tissue Release for the Lower Limbs

This chapter outlines how to apply soft tissue release to the lower limbs. Here you will find comparisons between applying passive, active-assisted and active STR to each of the major muscle groups of the lower body. Notice, however, that not all three versions of STR can be applied to all muscle groups (see table 7.1).

Table 7.1   Types of STR Used on Muscles of the Lower Limbs

	TYPE OF STR		
Muscle	Passive	Active-assisted	Active
Hamstrings	✓	✓	✓
Calf	✓	✓	✓
Foot	-	✓	✓
Quadriceps	-	✓	✓
Tibialis anterior	-	✓	-
Peroneals	-	✓	-
Gluteals	-	✓	-
Iliacus	-	✓	-

- **Passive STR:** Passive STR is excellent for treating the hamstrings and calf muscles. Technically, passive STR can be applied to the foot, tibialis anterior and peroneals but doing so may be damaging to a therapist's hands and thumbs. It may also be applied to the quadriceps but doing so is damaging to a therapist's lumbar spine. Illustrations of passive STR to these muscles have therefore not been included here. It is not possible to apply passive STR to the gluteals or to the iliacus.

- **Active-assisted STR**: As you can see from this table, you are able to apply active-assisted STR to all muscles of the lower limbs. However, that does not mean that you *should* use this technique for all muscles. Practice the technique to discover the muscles for which you find active-assisted STR easiest to apply.

■ *Active STR:* By using a tennis ball, it is possible to apply active STR to the tibialis anterior, peroneals and gluteals. Doing so is difficult, though, and may not be as effective as active-assisted STR to these muscles, so this technique has not been included for these muscles. It is not possible to apply active STR to the iliacus.

The following pages provide detailed instructions for applying passive, active-assisted or active STR to many of the muscles of the lower limbs, including tips to help you along the way.

Passive STR

Step 1: With your client in prone, passively shorten these muscles by flexing the client's knee. Lock the muscle close to its origin at the ischium. Each time you lock the fibres in this stretch, direct your pressure towards the ischium rather than perpendicularly.

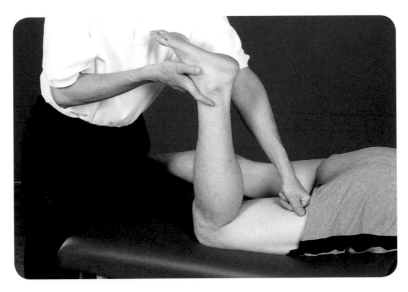

TIP You may want to explain to the client where the lock is going to be before beginning the treatment because locking under the buttock in this way may be considered invasive by some clients.

Step 2: Whilst maintaining your lock, gently stretch the muscle by extending the knee. Many clients do not feel much stretch at this point.

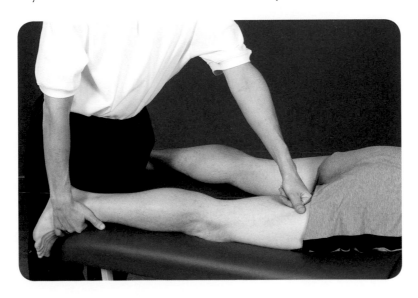

Step 3: Choose a new, slightly more distal lock, perhaps in the midline of the thigh.

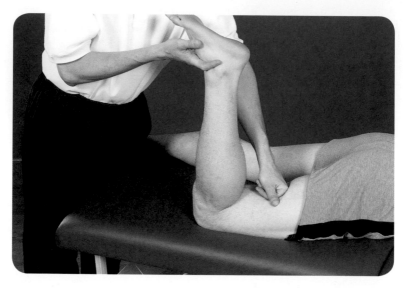

Step 4: Whilst maintaining your lock, stretch the tissues by passively extending the knee.

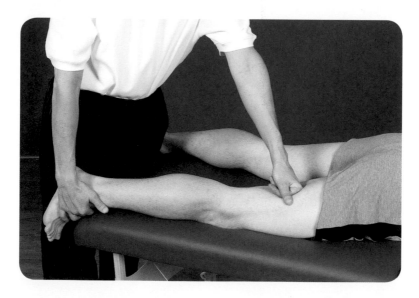

Step 5: Work down the length of the hamstrings from proximal to distal insertions, repeating this procedure. Avoid pressing into the popliteal space behind the knee. If you are performing the technique correctly, your client will experience an increasing sensation of stretch as you work towards the hamstring tendons. If your client does not feel the stretch, you will need to do active-assisted STR.

TIP STR can be used to help assess the pliability of hamstring muscles. Notice the resistance you feel as you work from proximal to distal on these muscles. Can you sense which muscles are tightest: the biceps femoris (laterally) or the semimembranosus and semitendinosus (medially)?

Advantages   Many clients report having tight hamstrings. This technique is helpful for assessing the pliability of hamstring muscles and identifying which muscles are tightest. ▪ Passive STR to the hamstrings may be incorporated into an overall massage treatment for the lower limbs with the client in prone.

Disadvantages   The hamstrings are strong, powerful muscles that require a firm lock to fix the tissues. Using a fist to lock the tissues is one method of locking, but this is not as powerful as using a forearm (as in active-assisted STR). ▪ When locking with a fist, make sure you keep the wrist in alignment: do not press through a flexed or extended wrist. ▪ It is tempting to use your thumbs to lock the tissues. Although this provides a great lock, it may be damaging to your thumbs. ▪ Elbows may be used to lock the tissues. Due to the length of the lever in this case, however, using the elbow makes passive flexion and extension of the knee difficult and may compromise your posture as you lean forward to lock the tissues.

Active-Assisted STR

Step 1: Whilst your client is in a prone position, ask him to flex his knee. Using your elbow, lock the hamstrings close to the ischium. Direct your pressure towards the buttock to take up some of the slack in soft tissues before the stretch.

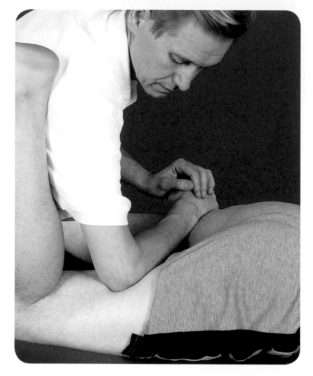

Step 2: Whilst maintaining your lock, ask your client to lower his leg back to the couch. Release your lock.

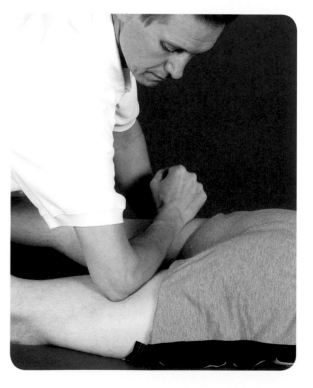

Step 3: Choose a new lock, more distal to the first. Repeat. Work in lines down the posterior thigh from the ischium to the hamstring tendons. Avoid pressing into the popliteal space behind the knee.

Advantages   This method allows you to lock using a forearm and thus provides a stronger fix to soft tissues. ▪ Active-assisted STR to the hamstrings is particularly useful as part of the rehabilitation process after surgery to the knee or immobilization of the knee joint. Using this technique helps increase range of motion at the knee and hamstring strength. Hamstrings contract concentrically each time the client actively flexes his or her knee; they contract eccentrically as the client lowers his or her knee. ▪ Note that the knee does not need to be fully flexed. When the technique is used after knee replacement surgery, for example, it may help increase knee flexion because the client works within his or her pain-free range.

Disadvantages   Constant active flexion of the knee may cause the client's hamstrings to cramp. ▪ When locking tissues, take care to guard your posture by taking a wide stance and ensuring that your upper-body weight is supported by the client or treatment couch. With practice, this is easy.

CLIENT TALK

Active-assisted STR has been great for treating a dancer who is flexible but nevertheless feels tightness in her muscles. I use client feedback to identify specific areas of tightness and work on and around those areas, sometimes with oil, sometimes without. It's not really possible to test the length of the hamstrings using the straight leg raise because this client can easily position her chest on her thighs before and after treatment!

Active STR

Step 1: Lie on your back, shorten the muscle by flexing your knee and place a tennis ball over part of your hamstring muscles.

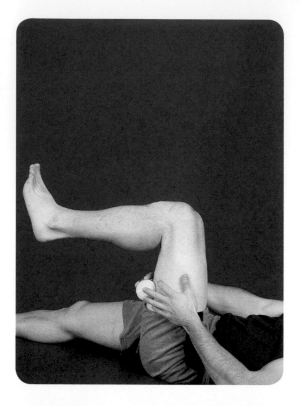

Step 2: Whilst holding the tennis ball as shown, gently extend your knee.

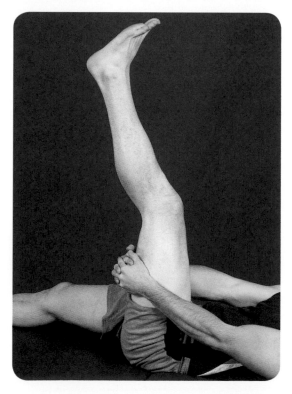

Place your first lock (using the ball) near the ischium and gradually work down towards your knee with subsequent locks. Because the hamstrings are a large muscle group, you will need to work all over them to fully benefit from the stretches. Sometimes it is best to work systematically, perhaps starting with the biceps femoris on the lateral side of the thigh, proximal to distal (ischium to knee). When you feel you have worked this enough, move your locks to a more medial position so that you are over the semimembranosus and the semitendinosus; continue to work this area in the same way.

You could also apply the technique in a sitting position if you were somewhere it was not appropriate to lie down (in an office, for example). Simply place the ball beneath your thigh whilst sitting so that it is between you and the chair, and then straighten your leg. Note, however, that this places considerably more pressure on your hamstrings and may be painful because you now have the weight of your thigh resting on the ball as you are sitting.

Advantage   The technique may be used when sitting and may therefore be useful for treating your hamstrings during the day if you have a desk job.

Disadvantages   If you have large, strong hamstrings, it may be difficult to apply the necessary amount of pressure to lock the tissues. ■ Conversely, active STR to the hamstrings when sitting places considerably more pressure on your hamstrings and could be painful.

Passive STR

Step 1: Position your client in prone with her feet off the end of the treatment couch.

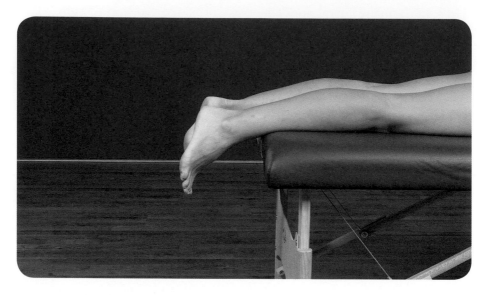

Step 2: Check that there are no clips on the edge of the treatment couch that may press into the client's foot. Make sure the client can dorsiflex at the ankle. One way to do this is to gently push the ankle into dorsiflexion.

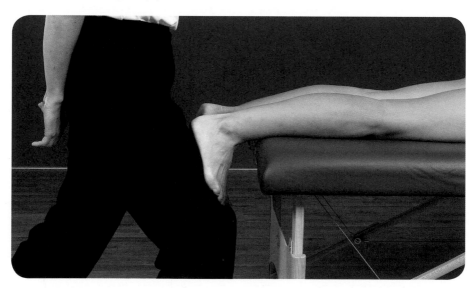

TIP Practice positioning your thigh on various aspects of your client's foot, either medially or laterally. Find the position that provides the client with the greatest stretch. When you apply this technique, you are going to need to provide passive dorsiflexion. Notice that to do this, you need to angle the client's foot so as to stretch the calf muscle, not simply press on the foot, thereby pushing the client up the treatment table.

Usually, it is best to shorten a muscle slightly before performing STR. The calf is an exception to this rule because the foot and ankle naturally fall into plantar flexion, where the muscles are already in neutral, neither stretched nor contracted.

Step 3: Whilst standing at the end of the couch, lock the calf using reinforced thumbs, just distal to the knee joint, perhaps in the centre of the calf. Each time you lock the fibres in this stretch, direct your pressure towards the knee rather than perpendicularly.

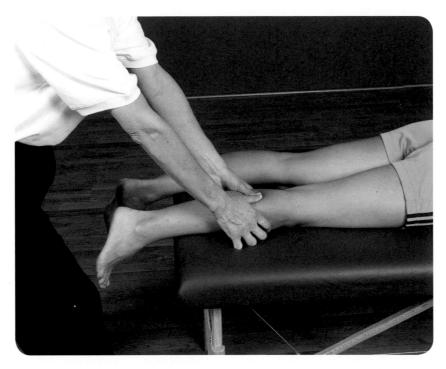

To demonstrate passive STR to the calf, this therapist has used reinforced thumbs. This approach is useful in working through the following steps until you get the hang of passive STR. However, it is essential for all therapists to protect their own limbs, and overuse of the thumbs should be avoided. Because they are plantar flexors, calf muscles are exceptionally strong, and it may be necessary to use a particularly firm lock when treating them. Although it may be tempting to press harder with your thumbs, this should be avoided. Once you have mastered the technique, practice using your elbow or forearm. Because this provides much deeper pressure and therefore a firmer lock, do get feedback from your client.

Step 4: Whilst maintaining your lock, use your thigh to dorsiflex the client's ankle.

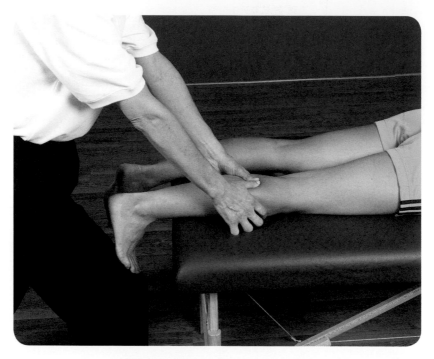

Step 5: Once you have dorsiflexed the ankle, release your lock, remove your thigh and move to a new locking position distal to your first lock.

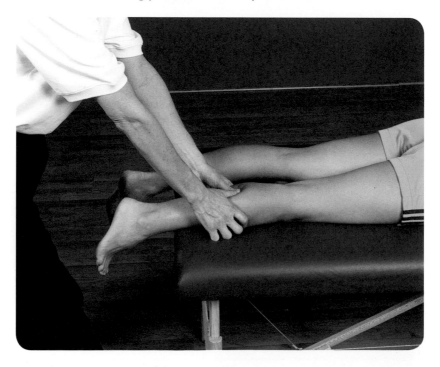

Step 6: Dorsiflex the ankle once again.

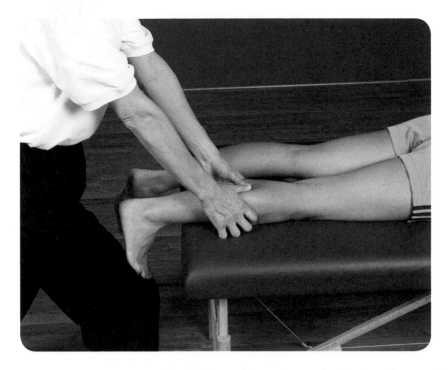

Step 7: Once you have dorsiflexed the ankle, release the lock and your thigh, then place a new, more distal lock.

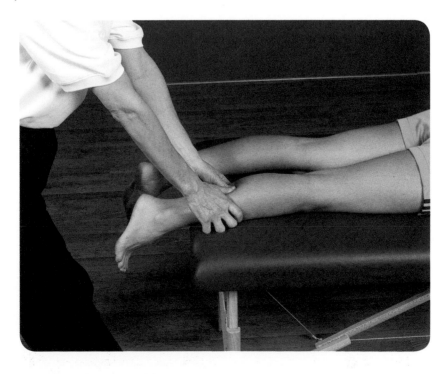

Step 8: Once again, passively dorsiflex the ankle.

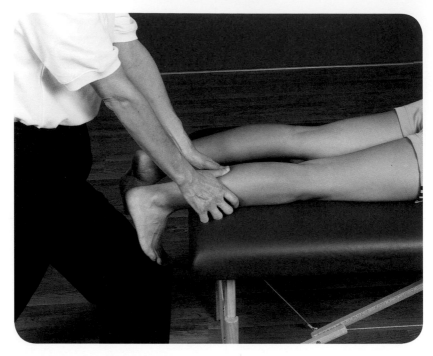

Step 9: Work down the length of the muscle proximally to the junction of the muscle with its Achilles tendon. Repeat this along the same line of the calf up to three times.

TIP The gastrocnemius, the most superficial calf muscle, is a bipennate muscle, with two bellies. Once you have performed STR down the centre of the muscle, move to the lateral belly and work this in the same way. Notice that many clients have a palpable band of tension running down their lateral calf. Could this be thickened fascia between the lateral and posterior compartments of the leg?

It does not matter whether you start STR in the centre of the calf or to the lateral or medial side. Usually, STR applied approximately three times to one group of muscle fibres is adequate to help stretch these fibres and increase range of motion at a joint.

Advantages   Using the thigh to dorsiflex the client's ankle can provide a pleasant stretch in addition to that provided by the STR. ■ This stretch may be incorporated into an overall massage treatment for the lower limbs with the client in prone.

Disadvantages   Take great care not to overwork your thumbs. ■ Clients with large, bulky muscles will not necessarily feel the stretch because the lock required will need to be more firm than can safely be applied using the thumbs.

Active-Assisted STR

Step 1: With your client positioned as shown, lock the calf muscle using either your forearm or elbow. Place your first lock just inferior to the knee joint, taking care not to press into the popliteal space at the back of the knee.

   Notice that the muscle naturally falls into a neutral position with the client in prone and therefore does not need to be actively shortened.

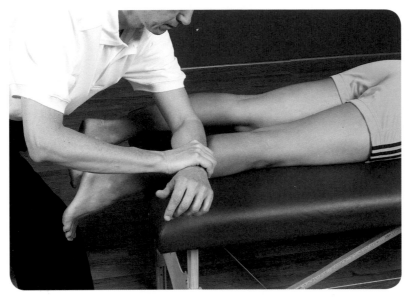

Locking the calf with the forearm.

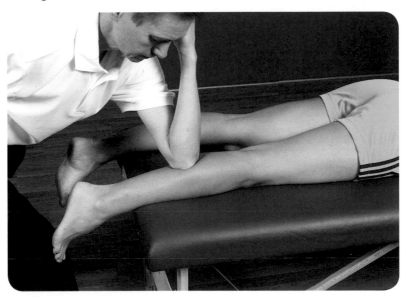

Locking the calf with the elbow.

Step 2: Whilst maintaining your lock, ask your client to pull up her toes, thus dorsiflexing the foot and ankle. Once she has done so, remove your lock and move to a new position.

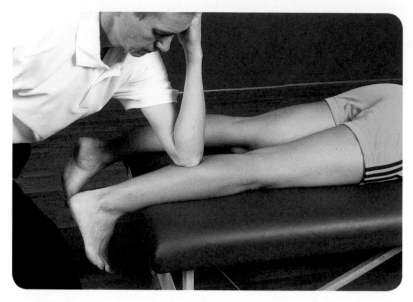

Step 3: Repeat. Work down the calf towards the ankle, stopping when you reach the Achilles tendon. Repeat in lines from the proximal to the distal ends of the muscle.

Limit the time you spend on active-assisted STR to the calf because constant dorsiflexion fatigues the tibialis anterior muscle. When working on a client after injury to the Achilles, the client is unlikely to dorsiflex beyond his or her pain-free range and is therefore not likely to damage tissues through overstretching.

TIP Make sure you transfer your weight to the client or to the couch: unsupported flexion of the trunk can cause backache.

When used with permission from medical personnel, this is a great technique to incorporate as part of the rehabilitation process after Achilles tendon surgery.

Advantages   This method enables you to apply a firm lock. ▪ Not having to stand at the foot of the treatment table means you can focus the lock in a variety of ways. ▪ The client is likely to dorsiflex to a greater extent than would be produced through passive STR to the calf and may therefore experience a greater stretch.

Disadvantages   Constant dorsiflexion will eventually fatigue the tibialis anterior. ▪ When leaning forward to lock using a forearm or elbow, be careful to avoid possible injury to your lumbar spine. Make sure you transfer your weight to the client or to the couch.

Active STR

Step 1: Place your calf on a ball as shown.

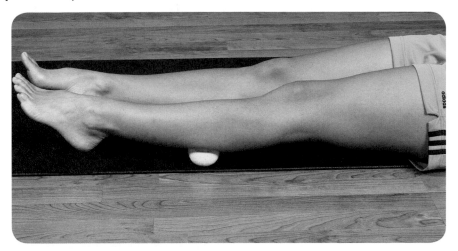

Step 2: Gently dorsiflex your ankle.

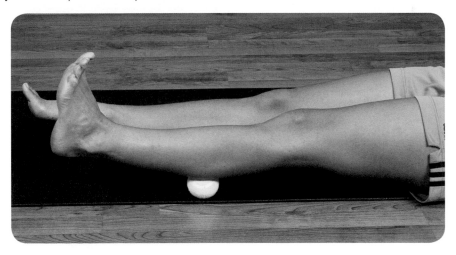

To shorten the calf, you would normally plantar-flex. However, you will find that your ankle falls naturally into plantar flexion in this position. Depending on how well developed your muscles are, it can be tricky keeping your leg on the ball in this position. An alternative would be to place your leg on a cylinder, such as a can, and apply the stretch.

Advantage   This is a useful technique for overcoming cramping in an acute situation.

Disadvantage   This technique places considerable pressure on the calf muscles and may not be tolerable for all clients.

Active-Assisted STR

Step 1: Position your client with his feet off the couch as shown; with the ankle in a neutral position, apply a gentle lock using a massage tool.

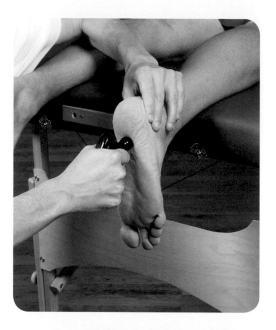

Step 2: Ask your client to pull up his toes, thus dorsiflexing the ankle and extending the toes. Work over the sole of each foot for a few minutes only.

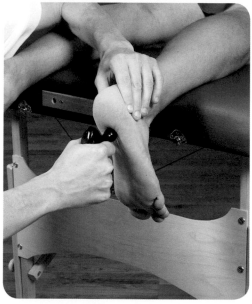

Advantages   Using a tool protects your thumbs. ▪ This technique may be incorporated into an overall massage treatment for the lower limbs with the client in prone.

Disadvantages   Not all clients like the sensation of the massage tool. ▪ Great care must be taken to avoid making too firm a lock. ▪ It can be difficult to get leverage here.

CLIENT TALK

A client trying to lose weight by walking to work started to experience foot pain when he changed from wearing training shoes to noncushioned flat-soled shoes. Having ruled out any serious pathology, I provided foot and calf massage on the client. He enjoyed the application of pressure to the soles of his feet, which I performed using a massage tool through a piece of tissue in order to get a secure lock.

Active STR

Step 1: Whilst sitting down, place your foot on a tennis ball or spiky therapy ball with your ankle in neutral.

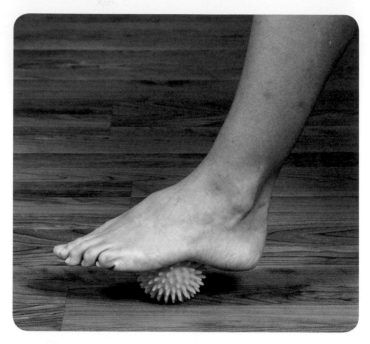

Step 2: Gently extend your toes, dorsiflexing your ankle.

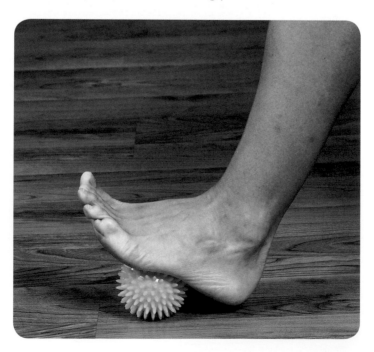

Step 3: Work over the sole, moving the ball to discover which aspects of the fascia are tight and would benefit most from the stretch.

Notice that in this instance you do not need to shorten the soft tissues. To do this, you would need to flex your toes, and many people find this causes cramping.

Applying STR to the sole of the foot stimulates circulation and has been reported to help alleviate pain in people suffering from plantar fasciitis. It is particularly good if you have had to stand for long periods of time or if you simply want to stretch out the plantar fascia after exercise such as running or walking. It is also great for helping to alleviate cramps in the foot muscles.

TIP When working the plantar surface of the foot, it is also useful to treat the calf because some of the calf muscles (flexor hallucis longus, for example) extend down into the toes. Stretching the calf may help ease foot pain in some cases.

Advantages   This active stretch is a quick fix for clients who have been standing for long periods or need to alleviate cramps in the foot muscles. ▪ The massage tool is easily portable.

Disadvantage   Care must be taken not to stand on the ball or overuse the technique.

CLIENT TALK

A client serving in the military police was suffering from plantar fasciitis in his right foot; he wanted to find a way to stimulate recovery because he had already had the condition in his other foot and found it debilitating. He was anxious that active-assisted STR might be painful and preferred to carry out his own STR, which he did successfully, using a golf ball instead of a spiky ball, over a period of weeks. Deep massage to the calf was used in helping alleviate tension in the connecting fascia, the aim of which was to take pressure off the calcaneus and perhaps also off the plantar fascia.

Active-Assisted STR

Step 1: With your client sitting, lock the quadriceps with the client's knee in extension.

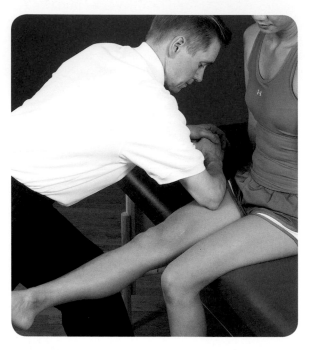

Step 2: Maintain your lock as your client flexes her knee.

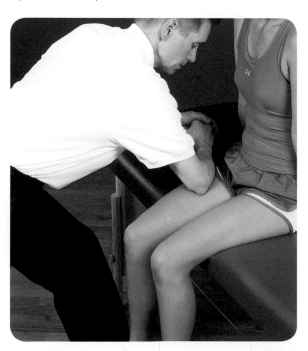

Step 3: Once the knee is flexed, release your lock and repeat, placing a new lock slightly more distal to the first. Work your way down the quadriceps from hip to knee.

Notice that the knee does not need to be fully flexed for the client to feel a stretch in the tissues. Practice locking the vastus lateralis and rectus femoris to locate areas of tension.

This is a particularly good stretch for clients who have anterior knee pain aggravated by tight quadriceps. Work slowly and carefully as you approach the distal end of the quadriceps; this increases the stretch and thus places greater pressure on the patella.

TIP This stretch can also be performed using your left arm to lock the client's right quadriceps. However, both you and the client may find this position slightly invasive.

Advantage You will be able to achieve a strong, broad lock on these powerful muscles.

Disadvantages Both you and the client may find this position slightly invasive.
- Take care not to compromise your posture. A wide stance needs to be used to prevent unsupported forward flexion of the lumbar spine.

Active STR With a Tennis Ball

Step 1: Lie face down on a mat; position a tennis ball beneath your thigh with your knee in extension.

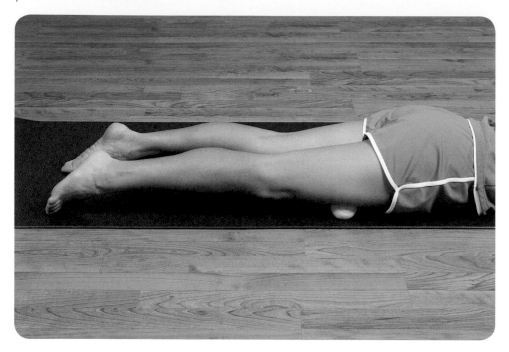

Step 2: Flex your knee.

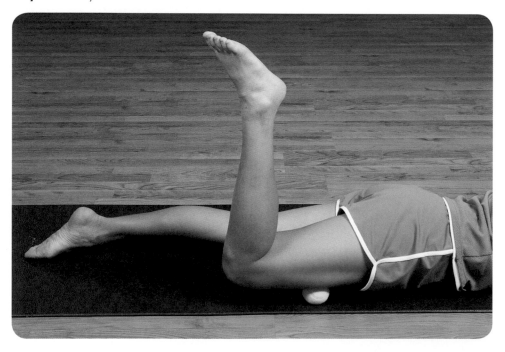

Practice positioning the ball against various parts of your thigh and notice where you most feel the stretch. Position the ball first near your hip; with subsequent locks, work towards your knee. To apply the stretch to your quadriceps, work systematically over this muscle group, from the vastus lateralis to the vastus medialis.

Advantage   This method is useful if you find that a general stretching programme for your quadriceps is not targeting specific tissues. For example, by positioning the ball to the lateral side of your thigh, you are more likely to access the vastus lateralis.

Disadvantage   Not everyone will feel comfortable in this position. This is a particularly powerful form of STR and may be uncomfortable for some.

This technique may be uncomfortable for some people because the leg's entire weight is on the tennis ball. An alternative method is to use a massage tool to lock into your own thigh whilst sitting with your leg in extension.

To apply STR actively to your quadriceps while sitting in a chair or on the edge of a massage table, simply extend the knee and fix your quadriceps using the Quad Nobber tool (see p. 17). Maintain your lock as you gently flex your knee. Repeat this several times on different parts of this muscle group.

Active-Assisted STR

For this stretch you will lock your client's tibialis anterior muscle. Sometimes this can be performed in supine. However, in this photograph, the therapist has positioned the client in side lying with her leg supported on a bolster in order to allow better access to the muscle. Notice that the therapist is supporting himself with his left hand on the treatment couch to avoid strain to his lower back.

Step 1: Locate the tibialis anterior by asking your client to pull up her toes. Whilst the client's ankle is in dorsiflexion, lock the muscle. The tibialis anterior is a strap-like muscle, and the therapist in this photograph has chosen to lock it gently using his elbow.

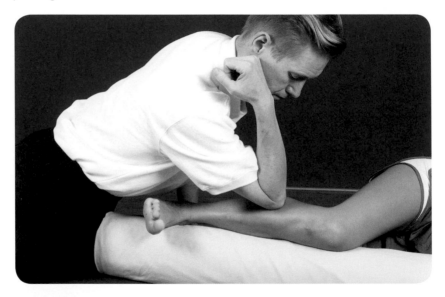

Step 2: Whilst maintaining your lock, ask your client to point her toes.

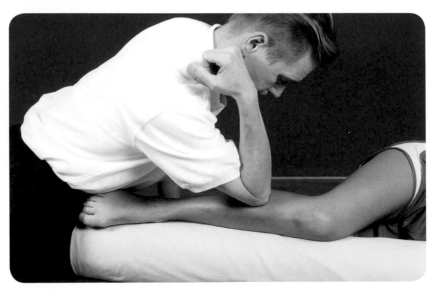

Step 3: Once the client has pointed her toes, release your lock and choose a new position, slightly more distal, for your second lock. With the ankle in dorsiflexion, lock in and repeat, working proximally to distally as long as the client feels the stretch and it is comfortable.

TIP The tibialis anterior becomes tendinous fairly quickly, so it is not necessary to work all the way down the length of the muscle to the ankle; to do so may be uncomfortable for the client because this muscle lies over the tibia.

Advantages It is extremely difficult to apply passive or active STR to this muscle group. ■ Active-assisted STR may be incorporated into a massage routine with the client in supine once you feel confident locating the muscle with the client in this position.

Disadvantages This method may compromise your thumbs if thumbs are used. ■ Avoid excessive pressure when using your elbow to lock the tissues.

CLIENT TALK

Active-assisted STR to the tibialis anterior was combined with an oil treatment for a client with shin splints. In an attempt to give up smoking, the client had taken up running; thinking he could train hard and fast, he had been running every day for three weeks until his activity was limited by anterior shin pain. Stress fractures were ruled out, and STR was included in a gentle massage routine twice a week for three weeks. After a period of rest, the client was able to return to a gentler running programme.

Active-Assisted STR

Step 1: With your client positioned in side lying, ask her to evert her foot (demonstrate what you mean). Lock the muscle, which is now in a shortened position. For demonstration purposes, the therapist in the picture has chosen to use reinforced thumbs to lock the muscle. Alternatively, use your elbow, remembering to be cautious to prevent bruising the tissue against the fibula.

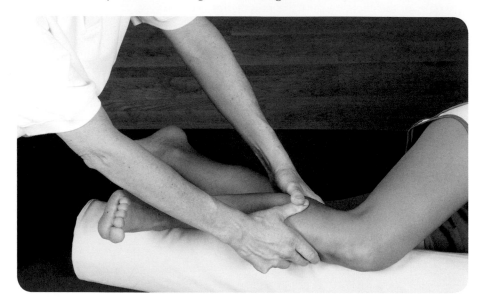

Step 2: Whilst maintaining your lock, ask the client to invert her foot (you may want to show the client how to do this first and, rather than using the term inversion, ask her to turn the sole of her foot inwards).

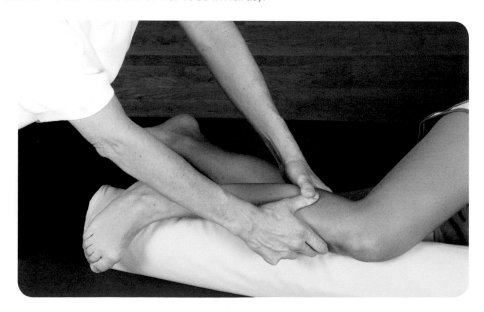

Step 3: Work in a single line down the muscle, from proximal to distal, as long as the client feels the stretch and remains comfortable.

TIP Clients with flat feet have particularly tight peroneals and may benefit from stretching these muscles.

Advantage   Active-assisted STR works best because it is extremely difficult to apply passive or active STR to this muscle group.

Disadvantages   This technique may compromise your thumbs if overused. ■ Avoid excessive pressure when using your elbow to lock the tissues.

Active-Assisted STR

Step 1: With your client in side lying, hip in neutral, use your forearm (close to the elbow) to lock the gluteals, directing your pressure towards the sacrum.

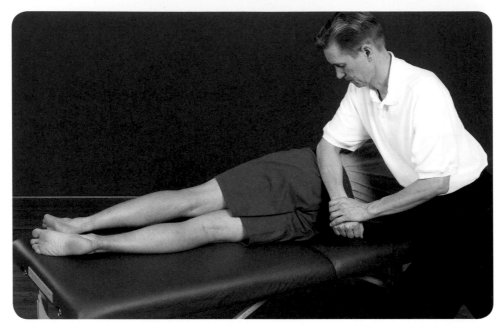

Step 2: Whilst maintaining your lock, ask your client to flex his hip (perhaps by asking him to take his knee to his chest).

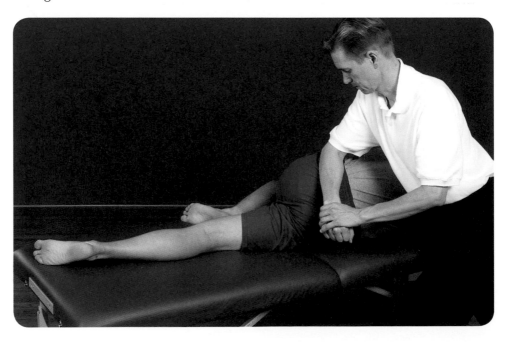

Step 3: Repeat this, varying the position of your lock, for a few minutes, working on the area that feels most beneficial for the client.

TIP It is quite challenging to apply active-assisted STR to the gluteals, and it takes practice to focus your lock in the correct spot on the muscles. With practice, however, you will discover that there is a small area that, when locked, provides for the greatest degree of stretch.

Advantage Active-assisted STR works best because it is difficult to apply passive or active STR to the gluteals.

Disadvantage It is challenging to focus your lock in the correct spot on the muscles.

Active-Assisted STR

This is an excellent stretch for clients with tight hip flexors. It is important to get client approval before performing this stretch. Show your client where you intend to place your hands.

Step 1: With your client positioned in side lying, hip flexed, lock into the iliacus on the anterior surface of the ileum.

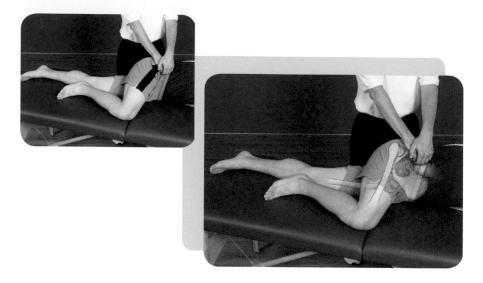

Step 2: Whilst maintaining your lock, ask your client to straighten his leg, which extends his hip.

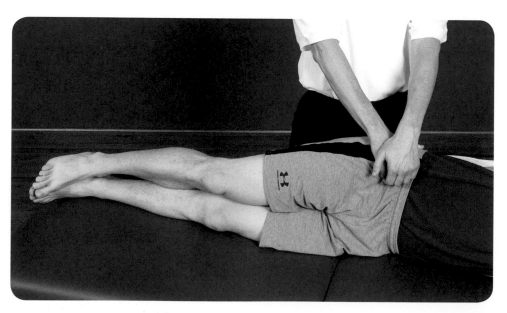

The area to be worked is small, so the lock may be repeated in the same place or a centimetre to one side. Usually, performing the stretch three times this way will provide some relief from tension in the hip area.

If the client requires a greater degree of stretch, rather than pressing more firmly with your fingers, have your client extend his or her hip at the end of the movement. One way to explain this is to ask the client to 'press into my fingers' when you get to the end of the movement.

TIP This area can be ticklish. An alternative is to ask the client to place his or her own hand on the area and then you press over it. Alternatively, dissipate your pressure by working through a facecloth folded into fourths.

Advantages   Active-assisted STR works best because it is extremely difficult to apply STR actively or passively to this area. ▪ The abdominal contents fall away in side lying, so having the client in this position is relatively safer than working with a client in supine.

Disadvantages   This technique requires a fairly strong grip. ▪ The area may be ticklish. ▪ Some clients may find the technique invasive.

CLIENT TALK

An office cleaner came for treatment for lower back pain. Tests revealed very tight hip flexors. The client frequently worked on her knees, in almost full hip flexion, causing shortening of her hip flexors and strain on her lumbar spine. After I explained the procedure using a miniature skeleton, I applied STR through her clothing over a period of four weeks to treat the iliacus. I also advised the client how to do active hip stretches.

Quick Questions

1. When performing STR to the hamstrings, which structure should you avoid locking into?

2. When performing passive STR to the calf, why do you use your thigh to dorsiflex the client's ankle?

3. Should you stand on a ball when performing active STR to the sole of your foot?

4. What sort of client might especially feel the stretch of STR to his or her peroneal muscles?

5. In which position do you treat iliacus: prone, supine or side lying?

Soft Tissue Release for the Upper Limbs

This chapter explains how to apply soft tissue release to the upper limbs. Here you will find comparisons between applying passive, active-assisted and active STR to each of the major muscle groups of the upper body. Notice however, that not all three versions of STR can be applied to all muscle groups (see table 8.1).

Table 8.1 Types of STR Used on Muscles of the Upper Limbs

Muscle	TYPE OF STR		
	Passive	Active-assisted	Active
Triceps	✓	-	✓
Biceps brachii	✓	-	✓
Wrist and finger extensors	✓	✓	✓
Wrist and finger flexors	✓	✓	✓

■ **Passive STR:** STR may be used passively on all muscles of the upper limbs.

■ **Active-assisted STR:** Active-assisted STR works well on the wrist flexors and extensors. Technically, the biceps brachii and the triceps could be stretched with active-assisted STR, but because the locks required are gentle, these muscles are usually stretched either passively or actively. For that reason, illustrations of active-assisted STR to these muscles have not been included here.

■ **Active STR:** All the muscles of the upper limbs may be stretched using active STR.

The following pages provide detailed instructions for applying passive, active-assisted or active STR to many of the muscles of the upper limbs, including tips that may help you apply the techniques.

Passive STR

Step 1: Position your client in prone and make sure she is able to flex at the elbow. Passively extend your client's elbow to shorten the muscle. Place your lock close to the origin, directing your pressure towards the shoulder.

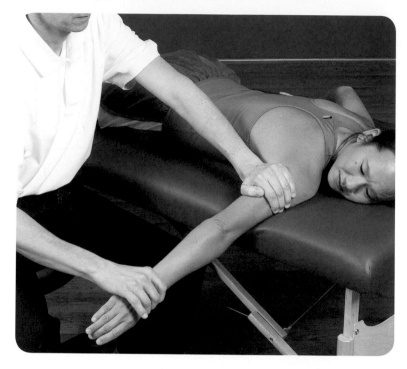

Step 2: Whilst maintaining your lock, gently flex the elbow.

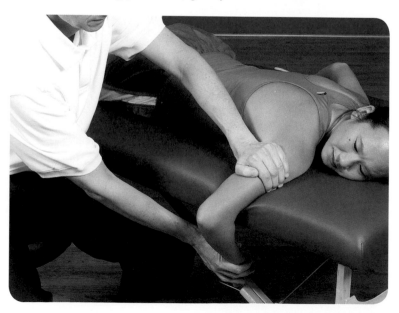

Step 3: Release your lock, extend the elbow and set a new fixing point more distal to the first. Repeat, working your way from the shoulder towards the distal end of the humerus. Your client should experience a greater stretch as you work towards the elbow.

Advantages   This stretch is easy to apply because the triceps do not need a very firm lock to stretch the tissues. ▪ By using a more specific lock, you can localize the stretch to particular tissues. ▪ Because you can use this technique with your client in prone, this is a relatively easy stretch to incorporate into a holistic massage.

Disadvantage   It may be necessary to move your client to ensure his or her arm is fully supported on the treatment couch.

Active STR

Step 1: Extend your arm and grip your triceps muscle.

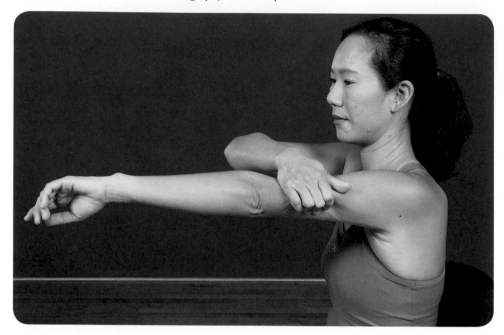

Step 2: Whilst maintaining your grip, gently flex your elbow.

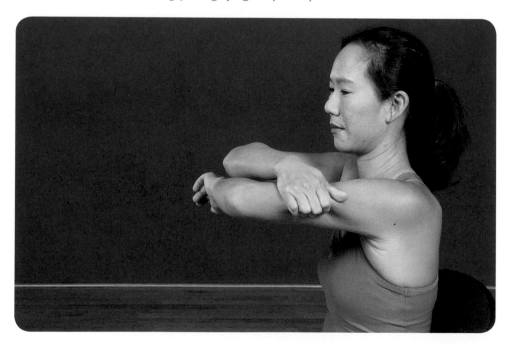

Some people do not feel the stretch in the triceps. However, most people will certainly feel it after activities involving prolonged or repeated elbow extension, such as tennis. Massage therapists who perform repetitive elbow extension when applying effleurage should practice active STR to the triceps between treating clients.

Advantage   This is an easy stretch to apply.

Disadvantages   It is difficult to apply a small lock actively, and therefore it is challenging to localize the stretch to specific tissues. ▪ When you direct your pressure towards the shoulder, you take up slack in the tissues and get a better stretch. However, when working the triceps, it is difficult to direct your pressure towards the shoulder; as a result, applying the stretch actively is not as effective as when it is applied passively.

Passive STR

Step 1: With your client in supine and his elbow passively flexed, lock in gently to the biceps brachii, taking up slack in the skin as you direct your pressure towards the armpit.

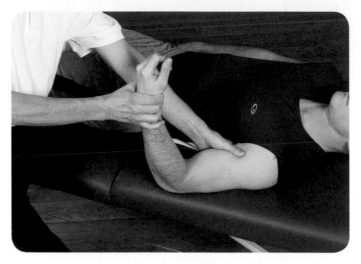

Step 2: Gently extend the elbow whilst maintaining your lock.

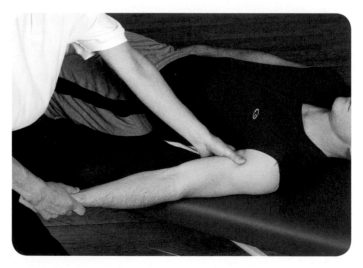

Step 3: Work from the proximal end of the muscle near the shoulder joint towards the elbow. Avoid pressure into the cubital fossa, at the anterior of the elbow.

Advantages   This is an easy form of STR to apply because the biceps do not usually require a firm lock. ▪ Because you can use this technique with your client in supine, this is a relatively easy stretch to incorporate into a holistic massage.

Disadvantage   It may be difficult to fix large, bulky biceps due to their cylindrical shape.

Active STR

Step 1: With your arm in flexion, gently grip your biceps muscle.

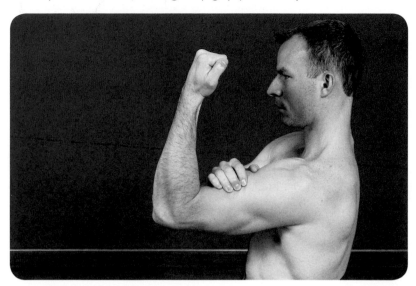

Step 2: Gently extend your elbow whilst maintaining your grip.

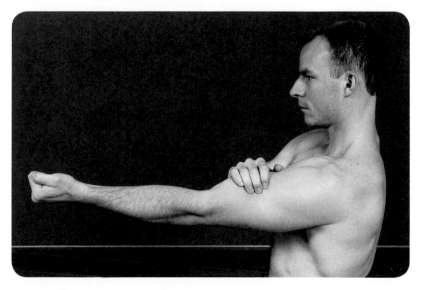

Applying STR to the biceps brachii feels good after any activity involving prolonged or repetitive elbow flexion, such as rowing, digging or carrying.

Advantage   This is an easy stretch to apply.

Disadvantages   It is difficult to apply a small lock actively; therefore, it is challenging to localize the stretch to specific tissues. ▪ It is difficult to direct your pressure towards the shoulder and take up slack in the tissues to get a better stretch.

Passive STR

Step 1: Gently extend your client's wrist. Lock into the bellies of the wrist and finger extensors on the lateral aspect of the forearm.

Step 2: Whilst maintaining your lock, gently flex the wrist.

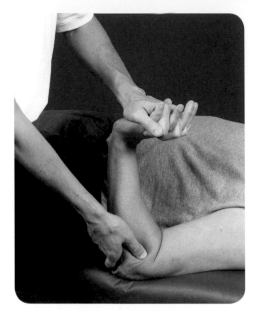 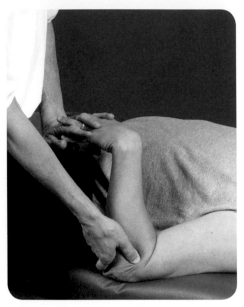

Step 3: Work down the forearm from elbow to wrist.

TIP To locate the muscle bellies, ask your client to actively extend his or her wrist as you palpate the area. You will feel the wrist and finger extensors contracting.

CLIENT TALK

Passive STR to the wrist and finger extensors was used in conjunction with a full upper-limb massage for a client recovering from lateral epicondylitis (tennis elbow) from playing tennis. The client was shown how to perform active STR herself in between treatment sessions, along with self-massage. She was advised not to apply active STR before playing tennis because to do so might decrease her grip strength.

Advantages   Because you can use this technique when your client is supine, this is a relatively easy stretch to incorporate into a holistic massage. ▪ Little pressure is required to lock the tissues.

Disadvantages   Getting the correct handhold so that you can flex and extend the wrist can be tricky when first learning the technique. ▪ It can be difficult to get leverage on the muscle bellies with your client in supine.

Active-Assisted STR

Step 1: Locate the bellies of the wrist and finger extensors by asking your client to extend his wrist. Lock the tissues.

Step 2: Whilst maintaining your lock, ask your client to flex his wrist.

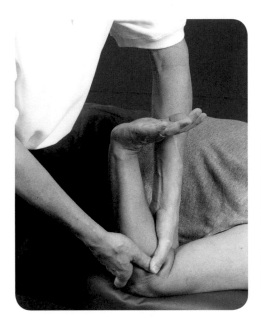 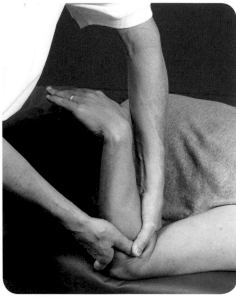

Step 3: Repeat the lock over the lateral aspect of the elbow where the muscle bellies are located.

TIP This is beneficial for the treatment of conditions such as lateral epicondylitis and for clients who perform repeated wrist extension, such as tennis players. However, the technique requires active wrist extension and therefore may fatigue those muscles.

Advantages You are able to apply slightly more pressure using reinforced thumbs. ■ Applying active-assisted STR is useful when working with clients who do not feel the stretch when it is performed passively.

Disadvantage It can be difficult to get leverage on the muscle bellies with your client in supine.

Active STR

Step 1: Locate the bellies of your wrist and finger extensor muscles. These are on the lateral posterior side of your forearm. Gently lock into the tissues with your wrist in extension.

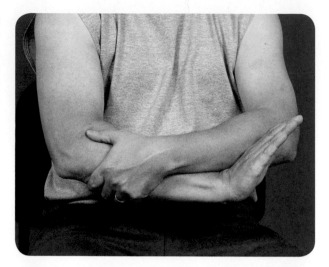

Step 2: Whilst maintaining your lock, gently flex your wrist.

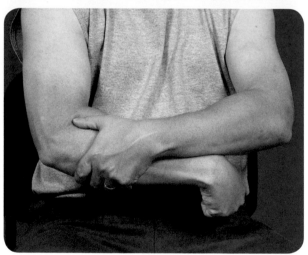

Step 3: Work all over your wrist extensors from proximal (near the elbow) to distal (near the wrist).

TIP Directing your pressure towards your elbow rather than perpendicularly into the muscle provides a better stretch. This is especially useful for typists, anyone suffering from tennis elbow and after activities involving gripping, such as carrying heavy bags.

Advantage This is a relatively easy stretch to apply. It is great for massage therapists to use on their own forearms between treating clients.

Disadvantage Care needs to be taken to avoid excess pressure on the thumbs.

Passive STR

Step 1: Ask your client to flex her wrist. Gently lock into the common flexor origin.

Step 2: Gently extend the client's wrist whilst maintaining your lock.

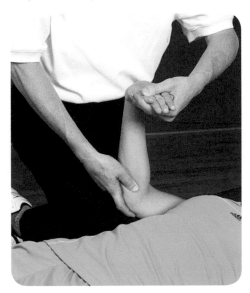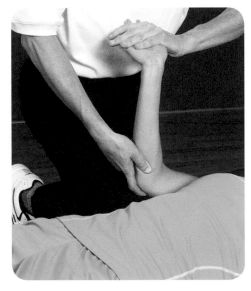

Step 3: Work down the forearm from proximal (elbow) to distal (wrist).

TIP To locate the muscle bellies, ask your client to actively flex her wrist as you palpate the area. You will feel the wrist and finger flexors contracting.

TIP You may find that it is better to work close to the origin of this muscle group, which quickly becomes tendinous in the forearm. Pressure into the anterior forearm is uncomfortable for some clients.

Advantage   Because you can use this technique when your client is in supine, this is a relatively easy stretch to incorporate into a holistic massage.

Disadvantages   Getting the correct handhold so that you can flex and extend the wrist can be tricky when first learning the technique. ▪ To fully stretch wrist and finger flexors, it is best if the fingers as well as the wrist are extended, as in the photographs shown here, but this can be a difficult manoeuvre when you are using one hand.

Active-Assisted STR

Step 1: Identify the muscles by asking the client to flex her wrist. Lock the tissues over the muscle bellies.

Step 2: Whilst maintaining your lock, ask your client to extend her wrist.

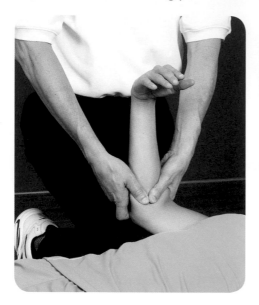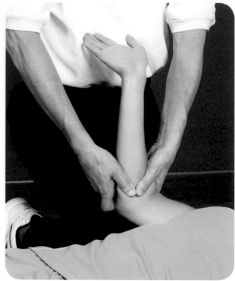

Step 3: Repeat this lock, stretch, lock, stretch sequence over the muscle bellies.

Advantages   You can apply slightly more pressure using reinforced thumbs. ▪ This technique is useful when working with clients who do not feel the stretch when it is performed passively.

Disadvantage   It can be difficult to get leverage on the muscle bellies with your client in supine.

Active STR

Step 1: Identify the bellies of your wrist and finger flexors. Do this by palpating your forearm on the anterior surface as you flex your wrist and fingers. You will discover the muscles on the medial aspect of the forearm. With your wrist in flexion, gently lock into this area, gently pulling the tissues towards the elbow.

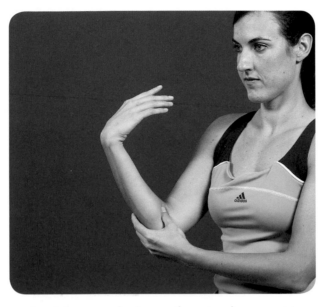

Step 2: Whilst maintaining your lock, gently extend your wrist.

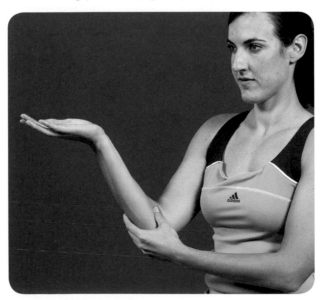

Step 3: Work your way from the elbow to the wrist.

TIP You may need to lessen your pressure as you work distally. This is because the forearm becomes stringy with tendons and contains many neural and vascular structures that may be compressed on the anterior surface.

This is a great stretch for typists, who are constantly flexing their fingers, and for drivers who, in gripping the steering wheel, are constantly working these muscles. It is also great for golfers and may alleviate the discomfort of golfer's elbow. Massage therapists who use their hands for applying petrissage should practice active STR to their wrist flexors between treating clients.

Advantage This is a relatively easy stretch to apply. It is great for massage therapists to use on their own forearms between treating clients.

Disadvantage Care needs to be taken to avoid excess pressure on the thumb.

CLIENT TALK

I frequently apply STR to my own wrist flexors if I have had to carry heavy shopping bags or treatment couches. I also used it whilst writing this book when taking breaks from typing.

Quick Questions

1. When are you particularly likely to feel STR in the triceps?
2. In which position is the client when receiving passive STR to the triceps?
3. When performing active STR to wrist extensors, do you start with your wrist in extension or flexion?
4. When performing active-assisted STR to wrist flexors, do you lock in near the elbow or near the wrist?
5. Give examples of three clients who might benefit from STR to the wrist flexors.

PART IV

Soft Tissue Release Programmes

This part of the book tells you all about the client consultation process, gives examples of the kinds of initial questions you might want to ask and provides examples of the types of documentation used by some therapists. Reading through the rationale behind the different consultation forms and comparing information from two very different case studies will give you a feel for how data are used to help design a treatment programme. Although therapists use different consultation forms to ensure they meet the requirements of their regulatory bodies and insurance agencies, those provided here are useful examples. How do they compare to your own forms? Do you ask similar questions to those listed in the Initial Questions section? Do you use a body map, for example, or a visual analogue scale? Overall, this section is intended to help you identify how a treatment programme might be put together. It is descriptive rather than prescriptive. Use it to help you incorporate STR into your own treatment programmes, amending the different sections of your consultation process as necessary.

Creating a Soft Tissue Release Programme

Every therapist knows the importance of consulting with his or her client. The therapist needs to find out the reason the client has sought treatment, what the client expects from the treatment and, perhaps most important, whether there are any factors that may contraindicate possible treatment. All sorts of forms are used to document information about the client, including body maps, on which the therapist (or the client) highlights symptoms, and visual analogue scales, used to record the intensity of pain, stiffness or some other sensation. Most governing bodies and insurance agencies insist that, as therapists, we not only document our treatments in detail, but also that our clients have consented to particular treatments and that we have taken reasonable steps to ensure that our treatment is not contraindicated. Most of you reading this will be familiar with these requirements and understand that they are beneficial for us all: they protect us as therapists, protect the client and help ensure and maintain our professionalism. Nevertheless, it is useful to review the rationale behind each of the consultation forms. You may find this especially helpful if you are a newly qualified therapist or practice bodywork other than massage and are interested in learning more about the differences or similarities between the forms used in massage consultations and forms with which you are already familiar.

We'll start by looking at some of the questions you might ask your client when he or she approaches you for the first treatment. As you read through these questions, you may want to tick off those you already ask and identify any that are new. Next, we'll look at the body map chart and a visual analogue scale (VAS), two methods of recording information. We'll also consider the value of carrying out a postural assessment, and consider why range of motion (ROM) and other special tests might be used. Finally we'll review two case studies and examine how the information that was gathered affected the overall treatment programme; we'll also provide examples of the full documentation used for one of these and summarise the other.

By the end of this chapter, you may have discovered some things you want to add to your own consultations. Perhaps you will simply feel reassured that the consultations you are currently carrying out are sufficient. Either way, you will be feeling confident and inspired to start practicing soft tissue release on yourself and your family, friends and, of course, clients.

Initial Questions

Your initial questions form part of your client consultation. The initial questions in figure 9.1 help the therapist identify the reason for treatment and help provide clues as to the kind of soft tissue release that might be used, whether it is likely to be effective or whether it should be used at all. Some therapists like to use guided questions; others prefer to allow the client to tell his or her story in a semi-structured way whilst the therapist identifies and attributes the answers. All therapists aim to ask open-ended rather than yes-or-no questions: open-ended questions tend to elicit more information. It is also good practice to record answers using the client's own words as far as possible and to avoid prompting. It is sometimes tempting to ask, *Where's the pain?* when a client may not have come to you with pain but with what they call *stiffness* or *something pulling*.

There is no doubt that asking questions is a skill and is perhaps the most important part of the consultation process: effective questioning sets the scene for what is to follow. Clients need to feel at ease enough to tell you their stories, and as a therapist, you need the confidence to identify and clarify salient comments whilst keeping the initial consultation to within manageable time limits without making the client feel rushed. You already may have discovered how these initial questions determine the professional relationship you have with a client: when asked sensitively, they can help you gain rapport; when asked brusquely, hurriedly or in an offhand manner, they can alienate a client.

In cases where there is a lot of information, it is often a good idea at the end of the initial question session to summarise your perception of the situation and state this to the client. For example, 'So just to be clear, you never had any leg problems before. A month ago you took up jogging and have since noticed a gradual increase in *achiness* in the front of your thighs. This achiness is uncomfortable when you stand up or when you sit on your heels but seems to go away within 24 hours if you rest. You copied some of the post-exercise stretches you found in a textbook for runners, but admit to not doing them very often. Now when you try to stretch, the front of your thighs hurts even more'. This gives the client the opportunity to clarify any points. Perhaps he or she was not clear in describing what happened; perhaps you misunderstood something. Sometimes hearing the story read back reminds the client of something he or she had forgotten all about. This is very common: 'Oh, I did get kicked in the thigh once. But that was ages ago. I'd forgotten all about that! I was playing football, and a boot went in my leg. It didn't bleed or anything; there was just this really big bruise, but it went away after a while. Could that have anything to do with it?'

INITIAL QUESTIONS

Client Name:	Date:

1. **How may I help?**

2. **Where is the discomfort you described?**

3. **When did it start?**

4. **How was it caused?**

5. **Is it getting better, worse or staying the same?**

6. **Does anything make it worse?**

7. **Does anything make it better?**

8. **Have you had previous treatment for this complaint? Was it helpful?**

9. **Have you had this condition before?**

10. **Have you had any previous injuries to the same area?**

11. **Can you describe the type of discomfort you are feeling?**

12. **How does this condition affect your work and leisure?**

13. **Is there anything else you think I need to know?**

Figure 9.1   Use these initial questions to identify the reason for treatment and to glean clues as to whether and how soft tissue release might be used.

From J. Johnson, 2009, *Soft Tissue Release* (Champaign, IL: Human Kinetics).

As you know, one of the reasons we tend to ask so many questions and aim to work holistically is that, whilst a client may present with a hip problem, for example, an injury in one area can affect other parts of the body. A client might not be aware of the relevance of an old injury and so may either have forgotten about it or may discount it entirely, thinking it not worth mentioning. If a client comes with shoulder pain, for example, the client may not think to mention that he or she has recently recovered from a whiplash injury. Unless the client knows about anatomy, he or she may not be aware that some of the muscles of the neck also affect the shoulder.

Therapists of all disciplines who work in hospital and clinic environments often become highly skilled in asking these initial questions because they are working with strict time slots. We learn to identify which answers require further investigation and which are less important. Often, we also learn what kind of client we are dealing with, and this informs how we treat him or her. For example, someone who exercises regularly and intensely and with the tendency to suffer overuse injuries will respond differently to being told he or she needs to rest than will someone who has only just started an exercise programme and is keen to take as much advice as possible to avoid injury. In rare cases, it sometimes becomes apparent during this early part of the consultation that a client needs to be referred. However you structure your consultation, by the end of the initial question session, you should have formed an opinion as to why the client has come to see you, what and where their problem is and whether there are any contraindications to you carrying out further assessment.

TIP Making accurate, succinct summary statements is a skill in itself. If you want to boost your confidence in this area, try this: Practice asking questions of a family member or friend, summarising what the person says. You need to find someone who has something that they might come to you with for therapy treatment. Practice asking questions and timing yourself to see how quickly you can identify the main problem, any contraindications and whether or not, after initial questioning, you may be able to help. Give yourself 20 minutes. Try again, giving yourself only 10 minutes. Are there key questions that you can identify from those you have asked that could have elicited the client's main issues in just 5 to 7 minutes had you asked them earlier in the interview?

CLIENT TALK

A client in considerable pain came to me for back massage. He had suffered a very unusual accident: He was taking part in an exercise programme that involved galloping on a horse around a circus ring. Whilst trying to grip the horse with his legs, a safety harness attached around his waist pulled him off the horse. Whilst telling me this story, he stood up with great difficulty and, lifting the back of his shirt, said, 'Look at this'. There were two very large bruises on either side of his lumbar spine. Clearly, this was an acute injury for which massage of any kind was contraindicated, and he was immediately referred.

Following are some of the questions you could use as part of your initial questioning session. They don't have to be asked in this order, and of course, you may want to modify this list. As you can see, they are useful questions to ask when the client comes to you with a specific injury or problem in a particular body part; however, many could be skipped if the client is coming for general maintenance massage, for example. These questions are those likely to be included in a consultation carried out by a massage therapist. Sports massage therapists, sports therapists, physiotherapists, osteopaths and chiropractors may choose to expand and adapt these questions. Here, we have assumed that the client is likely to need some form of massage, perhaps including soft tissue release.

1. How may I help?

There are many opening questions and, unfortunately, two of the most common are *Where's the pain?* and *So what's the problem?* Neither of these is advisable, even when said invitingly, because although they are specific, they are also prompts. First, a client may not have any pain; they may have stiffness or tightness or a niggle. It's best to let the client report how he or she feels before using the same terminology yourself (*A pulling feeling? Does it also pull when you look to the floor?*). Second, the client may not perceive his or her condition to be a problem at all. Many clients come for massage as part of a general maintenance programme. For example, runners may use it prophylactically to reduce the likelihood of developing problems associated with the iliotibial band; some weight trainers believe it helps reduce the likelihood of getting delayed onset muscle soreness.

Choose an opening question that works for you. If it feels corny asking, *What may I do for you?* or too harsh to ask, *So, why are you here?* try being deliberately vague: *Anna mentioned it was your knee. Is that right?* This first question does not necessarily lead to a protracted explanation; it could equally take you to the heart of the issue (*The physiotherapist says I have a frozen shoulder. She wasn't sure but said it was ok to try massage if I thought that might help*).

2. Where is the discomfort you described?

The opening question should help determine the client's main complaint and the part of the body it affects, or any other reason for seeking treatment. If the client is describing a problem relating to a muscle, you need to determine whether the whole muscle or part of it is the problem. Some therapists, therefore, like to have a separate question that specifically asks, *Where is the discomfort you described?* You might reword this for the situation—for example, *Can you show me where it hurts?* or *Do you feel the discomfort in the front of your knee or the back of it?* Soft tissue release can be used in stretching specific muscle fibres. Therefore, knowing that an old hamstring tear is in the biceps femoris, for example, is useful because it means you can later palpate and perhaps focus more on that hamstring with your treatment. Often, therapists will link this question to a body map (see figure 9.3, p. 140) by writing *See chart*, or will make a small sketch if there is space on the consultation form. After subsequent treatments, you can refer back to this section to see whether the initial site of discomfort (if there was one) has moved.

3. When did it start?

Here you are trying to establish whether there was a gradual or a sudden onset to the problem. Is the client describing an acute condition, perhaps an injury he or she has just received, such as a strained muscle, or is this condition something that happened some time ago? A calf muscle that was strained yesterday, for example, would be treated differently from a calf strain that occurred a week ago and is still causing problems. The more acute the strain, the less likely you are to apply STR. This question also helps identify overuse injuries. Overuse injuries such as tendinosis come on gradually and may be aggravated by repetitive activity. Often, a client cannot pinpoint when a condition started, yet his or her answers still provide clues as to whether the condition might be treated with STR: *It comes on at work, when I've been on the computer for four or five hours.*

4. How was it caused?

There is often a known cause for an injury (*I was running and then suddenly felt this sharp pain in my leg, and I couldn't run any more*), but with conditions such as sore muscles resulting from postural stress or overuse, the onset is so insidious that the client may not be able to identify the aggravating factor: *Nothing caused it. It just hurts when I drive. It's worse when there's lots of traffic, and I have to change gears a lot. Then my arm starts hurting as well as my shoulder.*

5. Is it getting better, getting worse, or staying the same?

Knowing how the condition behaves is especially useful within the context of STR. If a condition is getting worse, it could indicate that the client has an overuse condition that needs to be rested or that the client needs to be referred. Neither of these conditions should be treated with STR. On the other hand, if the client presents with tight hamstrings that seem to be getting tighter, this could indicate that STR would be beneficial.

6. Does anything make it worse?

Knowing what aggravates a condition is very helpful. Overuse injuries are aggravated by using the affected part. The answer to this question helps the therapist identify whether advising the client to rest and refrain from using that part of the body may be appropriate aftercare advice.

7. Does anything make it better?

Knowing alleviating factors is also useful. Clients who report that stretching helps ease pain, stiffness or discomfort may benefit from STR. Some therapists ask, *Is there is anything you can do yourself that alleviates the problem?* Sometimes the client will make a direct statement (*No. It only stops if I stop cycling; when I rub it, it feels better*) or will demonstrate a movement that he or she uses but cannot easily describe: *If I sit up straight like this it takes the pain away; sometimes I want to go like this. That seems to make it feel better for a bit.* Muscle tension is often alleviated by stretching and changing position, so clients who report that these movements help may be more likely candidates for STR than those whose conditions may not be related to soft tissues.

8. Have you had previous treatment for this complaint? Was it helpful?

Sometimes you will not need to ask this question because the client will already tell you: *Massage helps* or *When I saw the osteopath it was fine for a while* or *The woman in the gym fixed it last time.* You then can explore what the previous massage entailed, what the osteopath did or whether strengthening or stretching was used in the gym. If the client reports that he or she has had massage before and that it made the condition worse, it may be that you will be less likely to apply massage again. Conversely, the client may have had STR before and be able to tell you exactly where the therapist put his or her locks and how much it helped at the time.

9. Have you had this condition before?

If a client constantly suffers from a particular condition, it may mean he or she needs more regular treatment, or it may suggest that there is an underlying condition that needs addressing. Perhaps the client needs to alter his or her training routine. Surprisingly, clients sometimes repeat activities that bring about pain: *I always get shin splints when I run on hard ground*; *I only get the neck pain when I drive for four hours without a break and forget to do my stretches.*

10. Have you had any previous injuries to the same area?

Although not always relevant, this question sometimes helps get to the bottom of long-standing problems. For example, a build-up of new scar tissue on top of an old injury that already has its own scar tissue may lead to an area of stiffness that requires a longer and more specific period of STR treatment.

11. Can you describe the type of discomfort you are feeling?

Some therapists like to ask this kind of question early in the interview, and sometimes the client describes his or her pain, stiffness or discomfort long before you ask about it (*It just aches all the time when I'm writing*). Be careful to document what the client says without putting words in his or her mouth (*When I turn my head, it feels like something's getting squashed near my neck, here*). This is useful information and quite different from a statement such as *I have pain when I turn my head.* One of the best questions you can ask is *How does it feel?* If you treat the client, you will probably want to check in with him or her to see if you have been effective. You can then ask, for example, *Does it still feel like something's squashing when you turn your head?* Some therapists like to use a visual analogue scale (VAS) (see figure 9.4, p. 141) that measures the intensity of the client's feelings.

12. How does this condition affect your work and leisure?

This question provides all sorts of clues as to how quickly the client wants to recover if the STR is being used as part of rehabilitation (*Once I can fully bend my knee, the doctor says I can go back to work*), how stressed he or she may be feeling (*Everyone else is going. I feel like I'm letting the team down; If I could just do Thursday's match that would be great.*) or whether the problem is limiting performance (*I get worried that if I start to feel my hamstrings getting tight that I'm going to pull something. That happened last time, and I had to stop training for two weeks*.) Overall, this question may help identify how the client is likely to respond to treatment and what his or her treatment expectations are.

13. Is there anything else you think I need to know?

This is a vital ending question. We cannot possibly know everything about our clients; a client may respond with something very basic, such as *Yes, I can only stay 30 minutes today because my child minder's sick,* or something that may have a direct impact on treatment, but might not be picked up by the medical questionnaire: *I want to try this again, but when I had treatment from that other practitioner, I felt a bit dizzy when I got up.*

The ways clients respond to your initial questions provide a wealth of information that is not necessarily the result of direct questioning. For example, their answers may reveal how they feel about therapy, medical professionals or their own body, and their responses often highlight yet more questions you need to ask. How a client answers opening questions provides hints as to how you might proceed with other parts of the consultation.

Client's Medical History

Obviously, the client's medical history is of great importance; it not only helps us identify possible contributing factors to the problem for which the client hopes to be treated, but it also helps us screen for contraindications to massage. You can find an example of a medical history form in figure 9.2. Remember that contraindications to soft tissue release include easy bruising, thin skin and hypermobility syndromes. Other possible contraindications to massage or STR include recent physiological trauma, long-term steroid use, excessively high or low blood pressure, varicose veins, contagious skin disorders, heart problems, diabetes, osteoporosis and pulmonary oedema. In some of these situations, massage may be performed on some other parts of the body but not on the affected part. It is also important to remember that massage of any kind, including STR, is contraindicated in the first 12 weeks of pregnancy.

Assessments

A *body map* (figure 9.3) is a useful, quick reference to which the therapist may refer before providing further treatment and for recording changes. It is simply an outline of the body, showing front, back and sometimes side views, onto which you record the area of your client's symptoms. This is helpful because you can see quickly whether tightness in the calf extends down the length and breadth of the muscle, or whether it is localized to a particular region, such as the Achilles. Some therapists use different types of shading to indicate differences in sensation. Darker shading might represent increased pain or increased stiffness, for example. Body maps may also be used to indicate areas where there were old injuries or local contraindications (such as athlete's foot, for example). When symptoms relating to

MEDICAL HISTORY

Name:	Tel. no. (home):	Tel. no. (work):
Address:	Mobile no.:	Date of birth:

Dr's name/tel. no.:

Address:

Occupation:	Weight:	Height:
Current medication(s):	Referred?	
Recent operations or illnesses:	Pregnancy:	

Circulation problems: (heart, pulmonary oedema, high/low blood pressure, poor circulation)	
Respiratory system: (asthma, bronchitis, hay fever)	
Skin disorders: (dermatitis, eczema, sensitivity, fungal infections)	
Muscular or skeletal problems: (fibromyalgia, previous fractures)	
Neurological problems: (sciatica, epilepsy, migraine)	
Urinary problems: (cystitis, thrush, kidney problems)	
Immune system: (prone to colds, reduced immune status)	
Gynaecological problems: (PMT, menopause, HRT, irregular periods)	
Hormonal problems: (diabetes)	
Digestive problems: (indigestion, constipation, IBS)	
Stress-related or psychological problems: (depression, anxiety, panic attacks, mood swings)	

INDEMNITY: I confirm to the best of my knowledge that I have not withheld any information relevant to my treatment and that I understand and accept full responsibility for the treatment that I am given. I also agree that I have given the correct information as detailed on this form, and should inform the therapist should these circumstances change.

Client signature:_____

Therapist signature:_____ Date:_____

Figure 9.2 Every client should complete a medical history. From it, you will learn important information about the client, especially regarding contraindications for soft tissue release.

From J. Johnson, 2009, *Soft Tissue Release* (Champaign, IL: Human Kinetics).

several body parts need to be documented, some therapists like to indicate which is the main area, perhaps by using circled numbers (1), (2), (3), with (1) identifying the main area to be treated. As experienced therapists will know, a body map does not always show the area of treatment, for the area where symptoms are being felt is not necessarily the area at fault.

Sometimes it is helpful to fill in the body map whilst showing it to the client and having the client confirm that you have marked the correct area. Some therapists decide to mark their body maps during the initial questioning phase of the consultation to get an overall picture of where problems are and where they have occurred in the past. This is especially helpful if there are many areas to be treated or a complex history of injury. Others prefer to complete the map either whilst palpating the client or after an initial massage treatment during which tissues are assessed. Recording information as the client gives it to you obviously documents what the client says and is regarded as part of a subjective assessment, whereas recording your own findings from palpation or massage is a form of objective assessment. It may not matter which method you use, as long as you remain consistent.

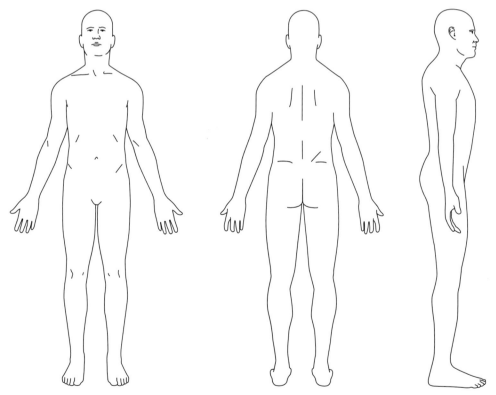

Figure 9.3 Use body maps such as these to record the area of your client's symptoms.

From J. Johnson, 2009, *Soft Tissue Release* (Champaign, IL: Human Kinetics).

TIP It is not always advisable to show your body map to the client after treatment if you are documenting your own objective findings. This is simply because you may find that you have marked all sorts of things all over the map, indicating where you found tissues to be particularly tight or areas of heat or increased sensitivity, for example. Seeing a body map covered with markings could alarm some clients, who might go away thinking that they have all sorts of things wrong with them, when in reality the map simply represents the subtle findings you have documented in a comprehensive manner.

A *visual analogue scale* (figure 9.4) may be used to document subjective measures, such as pain, stiffness, pulling sensation, soreness and others. The scales are quick, easy and effective. Simply draw a line on a piece of paper. At the far left end write 'no pain' or 'no stiffness'; at the far right of the line, write the opposite: 'worst pain ever' or 'maximum stiffness'. Show the line to your client and ask him or her to mark it to indicate symptom intensity. After treatment, you may want to ask the client to mark the line again, using a fresh VAS. If the aim of your treatment was to reduce pain, for example, the client's new mark should be more to the left of the line. It is not always necessary to retest your clients in this way immediately after treatment. Sometimes it will be obvious that the treatment has helped by what the client says and does. Also, long-standing conditions do not necessarily resolve in just one treatment session. Several may be needed before you want to retest your client using a VAS.

TIP Do not put numbers on your VAS. Clients remember numbers and may have a preference for a particular number. Or they may feel that they *should* feel a lot less stiff, for example, and so mark a 3, remembering that their previous mark was a 6. If you were to test a client using a blank VAS, you may discover that whilst he or she did feel less stiff after treatment, this was reduced to a 5 or even a 4, but not to a 3.

A quick *postural assessment* provides further information that may be relevant to the application of STR. Look for which of your client's muscles are short and tight and which are long and weak. Use STR to target the short, tight muscles, aiming to lengthen them, and avoid stretching the muscles that are already too long. Generally, when chest muscles (such as the pectoralis major) are tight, muscles of the thoracic spine (such as the middle fibres of the trapezius) are longer and weaker; when abdominals are weak, muscles of the lumbar spine (such as the erector spinae) and hip flexors (such as the psoas muscles) are tight. For more information on postural assessment, take a look at *Muscles: Testing and Function with Posture and Pain*, edited by Florence Peterson Kendall.

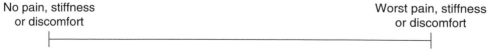

No pain, stiffness   Worst pain, stiffness
   or discomfort   or discomfort

Figure 9.4 A visual analogue scale.

From J. Johnson, 2009, *Soft Tissue Release* (Champaign, IL: Human Kinetics).

Range of Motion and Other Special Tests

If STR is being used to increase range of motion (ROM), then it may be useful to complete a chart highlighting the ROM of the joints relating to the area and muscles being treated. For example, if a client is being treated for tight or painful shoulders, knowing the ROM at the glenohumeral joint would be useful to assess limitations and to gauge the effectiveness of treatment. Other special tests include the straight leg raise (for hamstring length), the Thomas test (for hip flexor length), the Ober test (for tightness in the iliotibial band) and differentiation tests for tightness between the soleus and the gastrocnemius.

Programme for Treatment

Once you have gathered all the data, you will want to prepare a programme for treatment for the client. You can use a form such as the one in figure 9.5 to do this. Following is an explanation of the various fields on the form.

- *Subjective:* This section documents how the client feels and what he or she reports to you before treatment; it also documents that the client consents to treatment.

- *Objective:* These are your observations as a therapist. These include observations noted on the body map as well as data from the postural assessment, ROM, special tests and whatever you discover through palpation.

- *Treatment:* This includes a list of what you did and how you did it.

- *Assessment:* This section describes your assessment of the treatment carried out. Here you note plans to retest if necessary to see if you have met your treatment goals.

- *Plan:* In this section, you can respond to questions such as these: What do you intend to do for the next treatment session, and when is it to be? Is there any aftercare advice you need to give your client?

Case Studies

Following are assessments for two different clients, Client A and Client B. Take a look through them and then refer to their corresponding treatment plans. Can you see how the assessments helped influence the type of STR provided for each?

Client A

Client A presented with pain, stiffness and reduced ROM in the knee two weeks after being discharged from hospital following total knee replacement surgery. Client A's intake forms are shown in figures 9.6 to 9.9 on pages 149 to 152.

PROGRAMME FOR TREATMENT

Client Name: Date: /   /

Main problem:

Special notes:

Aims of treatment:

Subjective

Objective

Treatment

Assessment

Plan

Signature of client: _____

Figure 9.5   You can use a form such as this one to design a treatment programme for your client.

From J. Johnson, 2009, *Soft Tissue Release* (Champaign, IL: Human Kinetics).

CLIENT A'S INFORMATION   The following is a summary of Client A's intake forms:

- *Initial questions* (see figure 9.6, p. 149): From these initial questions, vital information was gained that helped shape the treatment programme. For example, the problem clearly affected the client's daily activities: she had difficulty going down stairs and was unable to walk her dog. Despite this, she may not have wanted to do her physiotherapy exercises because these aggravated her pain. We know however, that she is determined to get better: she is massaging her own knee and doing some of the mobilization exercises. It could be inferred that she wants some help in increasing her knee flexibility, perhaps by doing something less painful than the exercises she has been prescribed. We know that she likes walking and is used to regular exercise with her dog, which may prove to be an important motivating factor. The fact that she has had this operation before on the other knee suggests she is familiar with the rehabilitation process for this particular condition, although she may be frustrated at not recovering as quickly as last time.

- *Medical history* (see figure 9.7, p. 150): The main finding is that she has unmedicated high blood pressure. This is significant because after such surgery, there is often a period of recovery when the client is less active than usual and may gain weight; this often occurs with previously active clients, as in this case. Weight gain can increase blood pressure. It is therefore quite important that this client regains her mobility as soon as possible without too much exertion (exercise also increases blood pressure). Although the client has not reported feeling stressed, there is a hint of anxiety concerning the fact that her previous recovery seemed to be quicker. Stress can also increase blood pressure because tense muscles restrict capillary flow. The good news is that massage is believed to lower blood pressure, so it may be useful to use STR with massage.

- Also significant is that the client had successful total knee replacement surgery to her left knee two years ago. This suggests that she is aware of the rehabilitation process and may understand the importance of carrying out the physiotherapy exercises (despite not liking them). Even though massage therapists don't usually prescribe exercises, a massage therapist can sometimes play an important role in encouraging clients to carry out the exercise programme that has been set by the physiotherapist or clinical exercise trainer. Knowing that the client has been receiving treatment from another practitioner (a physiotherapist), it is important to gain approval for massage and STR. In certain cases, stretching could be counterproductive to an existing treatment, so it is always best to get permission and advice if necessary before starting a treatment. As you know, it is also a professional courtesy.

- Current medications include analgesics for knee pain. This is also important, for we need to know that a client can feel the depth of pressure of our locks, even when they are gentle, and any form of massage is contraindicated for clients who are taking painkillers of any kind. This also means that we need to warn the client that she should not take painkillers before treatment. This gives the client the opportunity to decline treatment should she feel the need to take painkillers. Nothing else was significant, and there were no contraindications to massage.

- *Body map* (see figure 9.8, p. 151). There is a longitudinal anterior scar on each knee. Using the map and medical history, it is easy to identify that the knee is the main problem area (though not necessarily the area to be treated), and that the scars represent surgical intervention. The right knee is visibly swollen. In addition to pain, this is likely to be a factor limiting flexibility.

- *Visual analogue scale* (see figure 9.8, p. 151). The client's main problem is pain, and she has marked a point corresponding to level 7 on a pain scale of 0 to 10, where 10 is the worst pain. This is quite a high pain score. It suggests careful management is needed, for although we do not know how irritable the knee is (that is, how quickly the pain comes on), we know that it is aggravated by weight bearing, so helping the client on and off the couch and not moving her about too much once she is on it may be important.

- *Postural assessment:* Client appears overweight. Scars support that the client has had knee operations. There are anterior longitudinal scars to both knees. Swelling to the right in anterior, posterior and lateral views indicates that the inflammatory process is active and that this may limit treatment.

- *Range of motion and other special tests:* Active and passive knee flexion were tested in sitting, supine and prone. All were uncomfortable, with flexion—both actively and passively—being the worst. The client preferred to have the ROM tests in prone despite having an anterior knee scar. This was an interesting and useful finding because it indicated that STR to the hamstrings could be performed with the client prone.

- *Palpation:* There was a slight soreness close to the scar but no other pain on palpation of the surrounding tissues.

CLIENT A'S PROGRAMME FOR TREATMENT   You can see the treatment programme that was designed for Client A in figure 9.9 on page 152. The main aim was to help the client gain an increase in right knee flexion and extension. Notice that although STR to the quadriceps could have been used, this was inadvisable due to the recent surgery. Therefore, STR was only applied to the hamstring muscles, increasing extension of the knee joint. As part of the treatment, the therapist gently increased the point to which the knee was flexed, distracting the client by gently shaking the limb. The overall effect was to gain 5 degrees flexion to the knee in prone and reduce feelings of discomfort at the back of the knee when the client was sitting with her legs outstretched, knee in extension.

The client was seen each day for five days initially, then once a week for three weeks. It is unusual for clients to come for treatment daily. However, this client was particularly keen to progress through her treatment quickly; because the treatment was light, not of long duration and resulted in an increased range of motion, albeit small, regular sessions seemed appropriate in this case. After five sessions, the client was advised to abstain from treatment, continue with self-massage and the physiotherapy exercises and apply cold to the knee if necessary.

Client B

Client B was a runner who came for treatment because his hamstrings and calves were feeling increasingly tight. Now that you have seen an example of different aspects of consultation, compare the Client A example with the information for this second client. The treatment programme (figure 9.10, p. 153) and summaries of the findings from the initial questions, medical questionnaire and assessments have been provided. Can you see how all the assessments help determine not only whether you use STR at all, but which form of STR might be used and how frequently?

CLIENT B'S INFORMATION   The following is a summary of Client B's intake forms.

- *Initial questions:* This client had started running four weeks before and had experienced increasing tightness in his hamstrings and calves. The feeling of stiffness came on gradually, as might be expected, and was getting worse. It is aggravated by running and sitting for long periods, and although initially alleviated by hot baths, now seems to be constant. Importantly, the client does not report any pain. The client may have pulled his hamstring muscle in a football match two years ago but cannot remember exactly when this happened. He has tried some stretches he found in a book, but they gave him a back ache. This seems like a straightforward case, with the treatment likely to be localized to the lower limbs. It may be worth taking a look at what sorts of stretches the client has been doing.

- *Medical history:* Client B suffers tension headaches (possibly related to his use of a computer for long hours), but there was nothing else significant and no contraindications to massage. Neck and shoulder tension can be treated with STR; this was noted for future reference but is not intended as part of this first treatment.

- *Body map:* The posterior of both lower limbs was shaded on this map, showing clearly where the main problem was. The fact that the client suffers tension headaches could have been noted on this map as a secondary problem.

- *Visual analogue scales:* Four visual analogue scales were used with this client to represent each of the lower limb muscles where he was experiencing stiffness (the hamstrings and calf on both the right and left leg). Interestingly, he reported a greater sensation of stiffness in the left hamstrings (5 on the scale), possibly where he had experienced a previous injury, and in the right calf (6 on the scale), perhaps because he is bearing more weight on his right side to compensate for the decreased functioning of the left hamstring. The VAS was 4 for the right hamstring and 4 for the left calf. It was noted, too, that the client's sensation of stiffness went all the way down to his Achilles tendon on both sides.

- *Postural assessment:* This revealed that Client B stood slightly slumped, possibly with a mild degree of knee flexion on both sides. Assessment was difficult because the client reported feeling 'uncomfortable' standing in an upright posture; standing with straight legs seemed to aggravate tension in the hamstrings.

- Because the client reported that he was seated at work all day, an observation of his seated posture was carried out. This revealed that he liked to sit with his knees flexed, his ankles hooked onto the base of the chair in a position he reported as 'very comfortable'.

- *Range of motion and other special tests:* The straight leg raise was used in testing the length of the client's hamstring muscles. Findings were 70 degrees on the left leg and 65 degrees on the right leg, with the client reporting an almost immediate increase in tension on both sides during the test. This was expected given that the client sits in knee flexion for about six hours a day at work.

- A differentiation test was carried out with the client standing to test the gastrocnemius and soleus muscles. There was decreased dorsiflexion on both sides and a shortened soleus on the right.

- *Palpation:* This assessment was done without oil. There was increased tension in the hamstrings and the calf muscles on both sides. There was a palpable mass of what may be scar tissue in the belly of the left biceps femoris muscle, which supports the client's report of a possible earlier injury.

CLIENT B'S PROGRAMME FOR TREATMENT   Based on the information provided, a programme for treatment was designed for Client B (see figure 9.10, p. 153). The main aim of treatment was to decrease feelings of tension in the client's hamstring and calf muscles. Although a straight leg raise test was used in assessing hamstring length, and this improved disproportionately after treatment of both sides, increasing hamstring length was not the main aim of the treatment. The VAS scale was used to help the client report his feelings of muscle stiffness: his main concern was not to have longer hamstrings but to feel less stiff: he was worried that stiffness might prevent him from continuing with his new running programme.

This is a good example of how active STR might be applied effectively in addition to weekly massage. In this case, it was important to explain to the client the importance of avoiding active STR before running because active STR might decrease his muscle power. It was also important for him to be cautious about applying active STR too deeply immediately after a run: there may be initially masked micro tears in the muscle that could be made worse with the deep pressure of the tennis ball. Active hamstring and calf stretches were applied as an alternative to post-exercise STR.

The client was then seen once per week for four weeks, and similar treatments were carried out. Feelings of stiffness decreased in both lower limbs. Post-exercise stretching was encouraged, and it was suggested that the client take advice on his seated posture at work. Although findings for the straight leg raise did not alter much, there was a marked increase in ankle dorsiflexion, indicating increased flexibility in calf tissues.

Closing Remarks

You should now have a good understanding of the importance of asking initial questions, and you have learned how a variety of different assessments can be used to help inform your treatments. The two case studies illustrate two very different situations in which STR could help. Can you think of any of your own clients for whom STR might be appropriate? Hopefully this chapter has given you some insight into the variety of assessments you could be using with your clients and has inspired you to try some of them.

Quick Questions

1. When asking your initial questions, what could you say instead of *Where's the pain?*
2. If a client presents with more than one part of his or her body needing treatment, how might you quickly indicate in your records which area is the main area of treatment?
3. What does VAS stand for?
4. In the programme for treatment, what does the subjective information tell you?
5. In the programme for treatment, what does the objective information tell you?

INITIAL QUESTIONS

Client Name: Client A	Date:

1. How may I help?
Looking for pain relief. Hoping massage therapy will help.

2. Where is the discomfort you described?
Pain in right knee.

3. When did it start?
Following recent total knee replacement surgery to that side.

4. How was it caused?
As above.

5. Is it getting better, worse or staying the same?
Better—slowly.

6. Does anything make it worse?
Doing the physiotherapy exercises to encourage flexion/extension!

7. Does anything make it better?
Not doing the physiotherapy exercises! For self-management, the client uses painkillers; self-massage to whole of knee avoiding anterior wound; mobilization within pain-free range.

8. Have you had previous treatment for this complaint? Was it helpful?
No. However, left knee replaced two years ago and seemed to recover more quickly.

9. Have you had this condition before?
n/a

10. Have you had any previous injuries to the same area?
Severe osteoarthritis, hence total knee replacement operation.

11. Can you describe the type of discomfort you are feeling?
Pain (level 7 VAS) on active and passive movement of knee, especially flexion; stiffness.

12. How does this condition affect your work and leisure?
Unable to walk dog; difficulty in all daily activities involving walking/stairs.

13. Is there anything else you think I need to know?
Client reports pain as 'burning' when attempting physical therapy exercises; this changes to 'aching' after exercise and may last several hours.

Figure 9.6 Client A's initial responses to questions.

MEDICAL HISTORY

Name: Client A	Tel. no. (home):	Tel. no. (work):
Address:	Mobile no.:	Date of birth: May 1936

Dr's name/tel. no.:

Address:

Occupation: retired school cook	Weight: 70 kg	Height: 5'6" (168 cm)
Current medication(s): analgesics for post-op pain	Referred? no	
Recent operations or illnesses: total right knee replacement	Pregnancy:	

Circulation problems: (heart, pulmonary oedema, high/low blood pressure, poor circulation)	Unmedicated high blood pressure
Respiratory system: (asthma, bronchitis, hay fever)	none
Skin disorders: (dermatitis, eczema, sensitivity, fungal infections)	none
Muscular or skeletal problems: (fibromyalgia, previous fractures)	Stiffness and swelling in right knee following recent operation, with decreased range of motion
Neurological problems: (sciatica, epilepsy, migraine)	none
Urinary problems: (cystitis, thrush, kidney problems)	none
Immune system: (prone to colds, reduced immune status)	none
Gynaecological problems: (PMT, menopause, HRT, irregular periods)	none
Hormonal problems: (diabetes)	none
Digestive problems: (indigestion, constipation, IBS)	none
Stress-related or psychological problems: (depression, anxiety, panic attacks, mood swings)	none

INDEMNITY: I confirm to the best of my knowledge that I have not withheld any information relevant to my treatment and that I understand and accept full responsibility for the treatment that I am given. I also agree that I have given the correct information as detailed on this form, and should inform the therapist should these circumstances change.

Client signature:_____

Therapist signature:_____ Date:_____

Figure 9.7 Client A's medical history.

ASSESSMENTS FOR CLIENT A

Visual Analogue Scale

No pain, stiffness
or discomfort

Worst pain, stiffness
or discomfort

Body Map

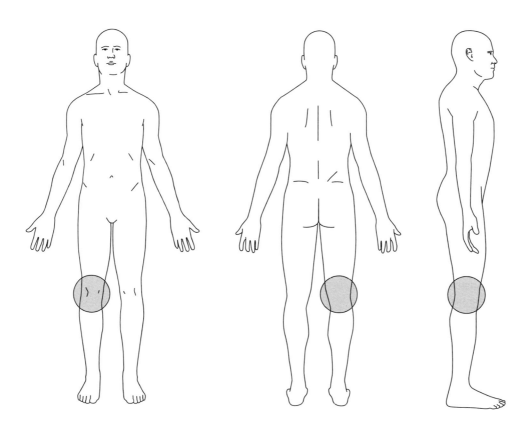

Figure 9.8 Client A's visual analogue scale and body map.

Chapter 1

1. STR targets specific areas of tension within a muscle, whereas general stretching works on the whole muscle.
2. You can lock a muscle using a forearm, fist, elbow or massage tool.
3. When applying a lock, start at the proximal end.
4. STR should be used cautiously in a pre-event setting because stretching temporarily decreases muscle power.
5. STR may be applied post-event but should not be too deep because there may be microtrauma, the sensation of which may be masked by an increased level of natural endorphins.

Chapter 2

1. You could use your palm to lock tissues when you need a gentle lock, such as when applying STR as a pre- or post-event treatment.
2. STR is not appropriate for the following kinds of clients:
   - Someone for whom general massage is contraindicated
   - Someone who bruises easily
   - Someone with hypermobility syndrome
3. The three types of STR are passive, active-assisted and active.
4. You do not hold a lock at the end of a stretch; once the tissues have stretched, you remove your lock.
5. To measure the effectiveness of STR you could
   - ask for feedback from the client regarding pain sensation before and after treatment;
   - use a visual analogue scale; and
   - do movement tests, such as the straight leg raise or prone knee bend.

Chapter 3

1. When a muscle is in a neutral position, the fibres are neither shortened too much nor stretched.
2. The therapist performs the stretch in passive STR.
3. Yes, a lock is maintained whilst a muscle is being stretched.

4. Clients are most likely to feel the stretch as you approach the distal end of the muscle.

5. You need to be careful when applying passive STR with oil massage because working through a towel onto skin that has been oiled provides an extremely firm lock.

Chapter 4

1. Both the client and the therapist work together to achieve active-assisted STR: The therapist provides the lock whilst the client moves to produce the stretch.

2. Active-assisted STR is useful for treating clients who find it difficult to relax during treatment and for those who like to be engaged with their treatment.

3. Active-assisted STR is a useful form of rehabilitation after joint immobilization because it increases joint range and helps strengthen surrounding muscles.

4. The biggest difference between passive and active-assisted STR is that in passive STR, the relaxed muscles are being stretched; in active-assisted STR, the muscle being stretched is often contracting eccentrically.

5. Some clients get confused if the therapist swops between passive and active-assisted STR because one requires them to move and one does not.

Chapter 5

1. You concentrically contract the muscle you want to work on in order to shorten it.

2. You contract the muscle first, then lock the soft tissues.

3. You place your first lock nearest to the origin of the muscle and work towards the distal end.

4. It is best to avoid STR if you bruise easily. Because it is necessary to apply fairly strong locks, these could induce unintentional bruising.

5. When you are first learning the technique, apply STR for only two to three minutes on the same area.

Chapter 6

1. In passive STR to the rhomboids, the scapula needs to protract in order to bring about the stretch. The arm, therefore, needs to be positioned off the couch at the start of the treatment.

2. To dissipate the pressure of any lock, work through a folded towel or face-cloth.

3. Active-assisted STR is a safe method of stretching tissues of the neck because the stretch is performed by the client himself or herself, and it is likely the client will stretch only within his or her pain-free range.

4. Be aware of the clavicle and acromion process and avoid pressing into these when applying active-assisted STR to the upper fibres of the trapezius.

5. Once you have locked the tissues to the erector spinae with the client in extension, the client flexes forward, thus bringing about a stretch.

Chapter 7

1. When treating hamstrings passively, avoid locking into the popliteal space behind the knee.

2. Ankle plantar flexors are very strong muscles, so it requires more force to dorsiflex the ankle passively and stretch those muscles. Using your thigh provides greater force and is safer for you than using your hand.

3. Never stand on a ball when performing active STR because doing so could be dangerous. Always apply the technique sitting down.

4. Clients with flat feet (that is, those whose ankles are everted) often feel STR to the peroneals more acutely than do other clients.

5. STR to the iliacus is applied with the client in side lying.

Chapter 8

1. STR to the triceps is felt particularly after activities that involve elbow extension, such as tennis, doing shoulder presses and polishing.

2. Passive STR to the triceps is performed with the client in prone and with his or her forearm off the couch.

3. When performing active STR to wrist extensors, start with your wrist in extension.

4. When performing active-assisted STR to wrist flexors, you lock in near the elbow.

5. Activities such as typing, driving and golf require wrist and finger flexion, and anyone who performs these activities is likely to benefit from STR to the wrist flexors.

Chapter 9

1. As an alternative to *Where's the pain?* you might ask *How does that feel?*

2. When a client presents with more than one part of the body needing treatment, one way to quickly indicate which area is the main area for treatment is to use a body map and mark the areas as (1), (2), (3) and so on, with (1) as the most important or main area.

3. VAS stands for visual analogue scale.

4. In the programme for treatment, the subjective information tells you what the client has said and how the client feels.

5. In the programme for treatment, the objective information records your observations as a therapist and includes information from the body map, postural assessment, ROM testing, special tests and whatever you discover on palpation.

Photo Index

PRONE

Passive STR

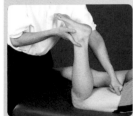 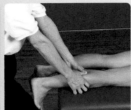 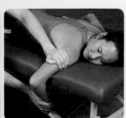 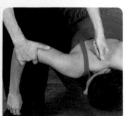

| Hamstrings | Calf | Triceps | Rhomboids |
| p. 81 | p. 88 | p. 114 | p. 65 |

Active-Assisted STR

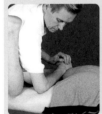 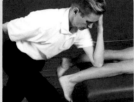 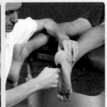

| Hamstrings | Calf | Foot |
| p. 84 | p. 93 | p. 96 |

Active STR

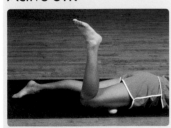

Quadriceps
p. 102

SUPINE

Passive STR

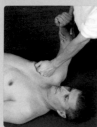

Pectorals
p. 69

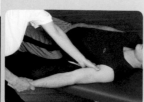

Biceps brachii
p. 118

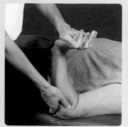

Wrist & finger extensors
p. 120

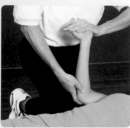

Wrist & finger flexors
p. 123

Active-Assisted STR

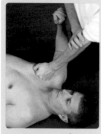

Pectorals
p. 71

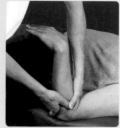

Wrist & finger extensors
p. 121

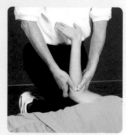

Wrist & finger flexors
p. 124

Active STR

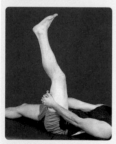

Hamstrings
p. 86

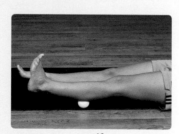

Calf
p. 95

SIDE LYING

Active-Assisted STR

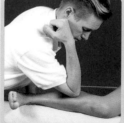

Tibialis anterior
p. 104

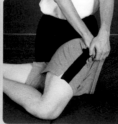

Iliacus
p. 110

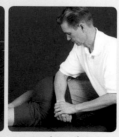

Gluteals
p. 108

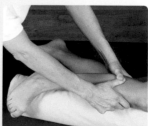

Peroneals
p. 106

160

SITTING

Passive STR

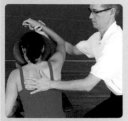

Rhomboids
p. 68

Active-Assisted STR

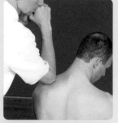

Levator scapulae
p. 72

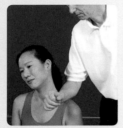

Upper trapezius
p. 74

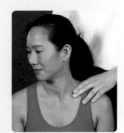

Scalenes
p. 76

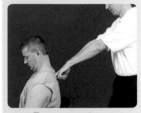

Erector spinae
p. 75

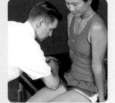

Quadriceps
p. 100

Active STR

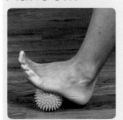

Foot
p. 98

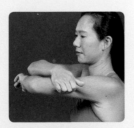

Triceps
p. 116

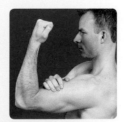

Biceps brachii
p. 119

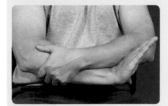

Wrist & finger extensors
p. 122

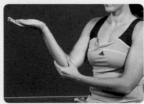

Wrist & finger flexors
p. 125

About the Author

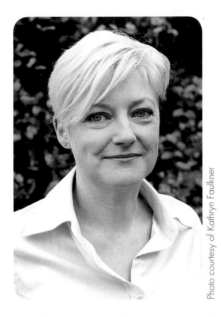

Photo courtesy of Kathryn Faulkner

Jane Johnson, MSc, is director of the London Massage Company in London, England. As a chartered physiotherapist and sports massage therapist, she has been using and teaching soft tissue release (STR) for many years and has a thorough grounding in anatomy, which she uses to explain STR in straightforward terms. She has worked with numerous client groups, including athletes, recreational exercisers, office workers and older adults; this experience has enabled her to adapt STR for various types of clients and provide tips for readers. Johnson has taught advanced massage skills for many years and has worked as a fitness instructor, massage therapist and physiotherapist. She frequently presents STR at conferences and exhibitions for therapists.

Johnson is a full member of the Chartered Society of Physiotherapists and is registered with the Health Professions Council. She is a consultant and examiner in sports massage for the Association of Physical and Natural Therapists and is a member of the Institute of Anatomical Sciences. In her leisure time, she enjoys writing articles and newsletters for therapists, taking her dog for long walks and visiting museums and exhibitions relating to human sciences.

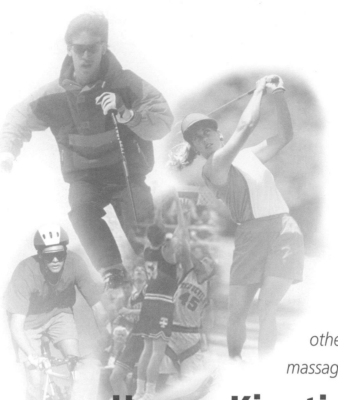

*You'll find
other outstanding
massage resources at*

www.HumanKinetics.com

United States	1-800-747-4457
Australia	08 8372 0999
Canada	1-800-465-7301
Europe	+44 (0) 113 255 5665
New Zealand	0064 9 448 1207

HUMAN KINETICS
The Information Leader in Physical Activity
P.O. Box 5076 • Champaign, IL 61825-5076 USA